TREATMENT FOR CHILDREN

Treatment for Children

THE WORK OF A CHILD GUIDANCE CLINIC

BY DAVID T. MACLAY M.D., D.P.M.

Consultant in Child Psychiatry Uffculme Clinic, Birmingham and Dudley, Hereford and West Bromwich Child Guidance Clinics

SCIENCE HOUSE, INC.
NEW YORK

All rights reserved. No part of this book may be reproduced
in any form without permission in writing from the publisher,
except by a reviewer who wishes to quote brief passages
in connection with a review.

© George Allen & Unwin Ltd. 1970

Library of Congress Catalog Card Number: 75-150530
Standard Book Number: 87668-040-6

Manufactured in the United States of America

Preface

The aim with which this essay has been written is to provide a handbook of treatment for the junior or trainee therapist working in a child guidance clinic. It does not aspire to be a complete treatise on the psychotherapy of children. For those who already have had a training in psychoanalysis it will provide few fresh insights. It is addressed to those child psychiatrists who are not analysts, to psychologists and social workers in child guidance clinics, to pediatricians, school medical officers and general practitioners who desire to undertake a measure of child therapy or who are forced to cope somehow with a case load of emotionally disturbed children. The probation officer of today and the child care officer of the future – they may be one and the same person eventually – will, I hope, find a good deal that is of value in its pages. For the benefit of such readers and for others who may have been led to work in this field I have tried to set out what I have learned during almost a quarter of a century of psychiatric practice and especially in the last sixteen years, during which time I have worked with children.

I owe a debt of gratitude to the many who have taught me, whether individually or by their writings, to my friend and colleague, Dr J. A. Crawford, who has kindly read the typescript and has made valuable comments, to my wife and our children who have borne the brunt of my too frequent detachment from family affairs and to my child patients and my grandchildren from whom I have learned much.

Dr Crawford does not fully share the optimism I have expressed in Chapter IV regarding the outcome for cases of *petit mal* – but I am satisfied that in our discussions with the parents of young children we need not give any gloomy prognosis. In the same chapter, where I have remarked that a school for deaf children will often be residential, Dr Crawford, with delightful imagination of the possibilities of day schools for such children, has commented on what a pity this is.

I wish also to thank Mrs M. A. Conium, S.R.N., for her contribution of a series of social work interviews in Chapter II and for her help in reading a large part of the text, and I am indebted to Mr David Bilbey for his account of the function of residential schools in Chapter XIII.

The first three chapters deal with our general approach to treatment. The fourth concerns nervous illness that is constitutionally determined, while Chapters V to IX treat emotional illness from the point of view of diagnostic categories. This is not to suggest that diagnosis in the narrow sense of putting a label to a problem is the best, or even a good, basis for therapy, but I believe that diagnostic signals serve a purpose for anyone who is trying to find his bearings in his search for meanings throughout the whole field of enquiry into childhood neurosis. Chapter X is an introduction to the techniques of play therapy based on the stage of the child's development, and Chapters XI and XII deal with the various techniques we employ. Finally, Chapters XIV to XVI are in some sense an expansion of the principles dealt with in Chapter X, as they are concerned with the therapy of children based upon the age of the child or young person from the pre-school years until after the age of leaving school.

A critic has commented that too little information is given on family psychiatry. In explanation I would say that family psychiatry is not a recent discovery or a new process, but is a name that has been given to an important aspect of child psychiatry which has been recognized and practised by children's psychiatrists already for a number of years. In Chapter II I have laid stress on the importance of influences within the family, while that it is an essential condition of the success of our work that we should integrate the togetherness of all the members of the family is implied in much that is said in following pages. The importance of interpersonal relationships within the family stands out from much of the clinical material quoted. Yet family psychiatry is not the whole of child guidance, because the child has also his own inner life – the psychology of hidden feelings within and about himself – and in later childhood he must also deal with concerns which are outside his family in the world of his social associations both at school and externally.

David T. Maclay
Barnt Green, Worcestershire, 1969

Contents

PREFACE		Page 7
I	Diagnosis	11
II	Environmental Factors in Diagnosis and in Treatment	19
III	The Unconscious Origin of Neurosis	31
IV	Emotional Illness that is Constitutionally or Organically Determined	51
V	Disturbances Characterized by Free-floating Anxiety	64
VI	Psychosomatic Illness and Emotion-linked Bodily States	78
VII	Problems Related to Education	96
VIII	Behaviour Disorders and Delinquency	112
IX	Problems Involving Sexual Development, the Integrity of the Family and Social Integration	124
X	Introductory Considerations to Play Therapy Techniques	132
XI	Techniques of Play Therapy	141
XII	Painting and Blackboard Drawing	153
XIII	Treatment through Relationship Formation	166
XIV	Some Typical Treatment Cases: the Pre-school Years and the Early Years at School	178
XV	The Middle School Years	196
XVI	The Later School Years and School Leavers	218
FOR FURTHER READING		236
NOTES		237
INDEX		241

CHAPTER I

Diagnosis

Understanding of the child's problem and of the emotional situation in which he is, is the key to successful therapy. Without understanding treatment must be hit or miss, but if we do comprehend we can treat rationally, or in some cases we may thereby appreciate that only a limited régime of treatment is appropriate. It thus follows that the first objective of treatment sessions is an understanding of the child's difficulties.

When a boy or girl is referred to the child guidance clinic it is our immediate aim to make a diagnosis of the problem, a diagnosis which is careful, which is comprehensive of the various facets of his history and environment, and which includes an assessment of etiology. Seldom, however, will this be a complete diagnosis, because it will rarely at this stage be possible to discover the exact pattern of the child's anxieties. This pattern, representing the nuclear problem which besets him, is likely to be apparent only in the light of the further study which treatment interviews will bring.

Sometimes, when after a detailed history and scrutiny of the circumstances there still is little to indicate how matters have gone wrong, one may be tempted to posit some constitutional element as being the underlying cause. The danger inherent in this will be that having assumed the existence of such a factor we may give up the determination to seek an explanation for the problem in the environment, in the child's relationships with parents and others and in the unconscious formations of his own psyche in the earliest years, or even months and weeks, of his life. On the other hand, so successful have been the teachings of Freud, and of those who have shown how destructive a faulty home environment can be to mental development, that some workers appear ready to insist that there must be an environmental cause even when such a conclusion is not in accord with realistic appraisal. It is, however, a cardinal feature of child psychiatry that we try to explain our children's problems on psychological grounds unless we can show that there is real substance in some constitutional factor.

Whoever has referred the child, be it family doctor, school medical officer, teacher, probation officer or someone else, will probably have provided comments and information which will be among the clues to what is amiss, but in the child guidance clinic our principal source of information at this stage is the social worker's report. The psychologist's findings also will be available and the child psychiatrist will have had an interview with the child himself and will have seen his mother. It is by a careful and imaginative scrutiny of all this information that an early diagnosis is made. At this stage we shall include an assessment of how the problem has arisen.

One of the chief difficulties facing the junior children's psychiatrist is the way symptoms have of being so divorced from sense. There often seems to be no reason to account for the symptoms and therefore no avenue to lead into therapeutic discussion. How does one begin to talk to a child whose hobby is cutting holes in his clothes? Are we to be surprised at the psychiatrist who wondered if behaviour therapy would be the answer for a boy in his early teens who had committed indecent assaults on girls? In adult psychiatry we have become used to the concept that symptoms often do not represent the reality needs of the patient. In child psychiatry our burden is no greater – we have to be able to see the child *in his environment*, to identify with him and to discover, in the case of a proportion though not all, of our young patients, what are the unconscious problems that are in need of expression. The symptoms can largely be disregarded.

The Social Worker's Report
It is appropriate here to consider the kind of factors for which the social worker will be on the look out at this stage. The child's place in the family and the age, sex and circumstances of brothers and sisters are a useful beginning; and she will go on to assess the degree to which the baby was wanted, the depth of love which dictated his mother's actions towards him and the nature of his father's care for both of them. She will try to discover what is the kind of emotional atmosphere which exists between the mother and the father, who else lives at home, what is the interplay of relatives in the life of this family, and what are the significant factors in the family especially as regards mental health. What was the mother's emotional state during pregnancy, did she look forward with joy to having this child and was she ready for the responsibilities of parenthood? The circumstances of the birth itself are important as bearing on the possibility of brain trauma from such causes as subclinical haemorrhage or anoxia. The mother's physical and emotional health during the puerperium, the degree to which she breast-fed her child, difficulties in feeding, sleeping or weaning, the nature of toilet training and the baby's

adjustment to life – was he happy, affectionate, compliant or demanding or did he cry excessively? – are important issues. The milestones of growth are important, especially when he first walked and talked, and it is useful to know when he became clean and dry, although the reflection of mother's attitudes implied in these issues can be their most important aspect. Illnesses are the subject of enquiry, especially gastro-enteritis and bronchitis in babyhood,[1] subsequent illnesses and any history of recurrent illnesses in childhood. Separations from mother or from the family during the first five and especially the first three years of life may be significant. The mother who develops a breast abscess during the puerperium may be unconsciously expressing anxiety, due perhaps to her fear that she will be unable to look after him.

The social worker will want to know of the baby's development within the family as he grew older, about his relationships with mother, father, brothers and sisters, about his ability to mix with other children and about his integration in school. She will attempt an appraisal, even if it is provisional at this stage, of the personalities of mother and father, of their capacities for loving, of their abilities to give of themselves and their time and attention to their children, or of any tendency to substitute material gifts for understanding love. The parents of the 'spoilt' child are those whose love lacks the depth of understanding that will impose necessary discipline – the child gets too much of his own way as compensation for having too little of his mother's selfgiving love, and when things inevitably go wrong the parent fails to shoulder responsibility for the outcome.

Diagnosis initially will be based on the history, the psychiatrist's examination of the child and his interview with the mother, and upon whatever physical examination has been undertaken by the family doctor or school medical officer or is requested of the pediatrician. In the vast majority of cases the diagnosis will be of some emotional disturbance and even in those cases where a physical lesion is present psychological difficulties are likely to be appreciable, and will influence therapy.

Physical Factors in Etiology
Especially in the case of younger children it is important to remember the influence of physical factors. In the realm of mental subnormality a number of physical causes are already known, such as cretinism, mongolism and phenylketonuria, as well as several congenital neurological disorders with which mental deficiency is associated, and a vista opens here of further discoveries and wider opportunities for treatment in the future.

In recent years, too, we have come to appreciate the importance of *brain damage*, whether due to pre-natal influences, birth trauma or subsequent disease, in causing emotional maladjustment, whether with or without intellectual impairment. This is not to consider cases of more gross damage such as may be due to maternal rubella, kernicterus or spastic disorder, but we are thinking of those lesser traumatic incidents which may previously have passed unnoticed because their effects could not be demonstrated physically and the symptoms of which have been regarded as due to some psychological cause.

An American study of 2,000 children has shown that a history of complications during pregnancy and delivery, especially pre-eclamptic toxaemia, may be associated with subsequent behaviour disorder at school, while some of the children developed tics, epilepsy or speech disorder and some were mentally retarded.[2] An Edinburgh study of 600 children gave similar results.[3] It has been suggested that it might not be toxins in the mother but foetal anoxia with minimal damage to the brain which caused these disturbances.

The Child's Constitutional Characteristics
One further factor of inherited endowment has to be considered, namely the strength or robustness of the baby's mental constitution. Some children appear to be naturally contented and able to accept frustration, while others demand more attention. Some children appear to thrive and to adapt from the moment of birth, while others have feeding difficulties, cry unduly or do not sleep well. There are again those who are predisposed to some disability which has both organic and emotional aspects, such as infantile eczema. When such anomalies of adjustment occur from the early days of life to the children of sound parents, or where one member of a family displays such qualities virtually from birth, while the other members do not, unless some activating factor can be adduced, it is difficult to avoid the conclusion that the problem is constitutional rather than environmental.

A child was referred by his family doctor to one of our clinics at the age of 2½ years, because of persistent disturbances, frequent outbursts of temper and disruptive behaviour. His mother gave as an example how, if she took him to a shop, he would insist on upsetting a stack of tins and fret for a long time if not allowed to do so. He was said to have been in poor condition for two days after birth and to have been given oxygen, and from the earliest days to have been a restless, 'edgy' child,: 'a "niggly" baby who would not sit in the pram like the others'. Development milestones were normal and he appeared to be intelligent. He was the middle one of three living children. The parents appeared to be happy and the family to be well integrated; the mother we regarded as loving and understanding, but she was under a good deal of strain, due, it seemed, to the boy's behaviour, and she wept in our initial interview. It was the child psychiatrist's opinion that this child had poor capacity for adaptation. Birth difficulties might be relevant, but we felt justified in postulating a constitutionally weak or inferior temperament.

The problem was discussed at length with the mother. The therapist felt they were just containing the situation, that there was an even chance that they would win through by existing methods of handling, and that it was best to let the child come into their bed at some time during the night when he wakened, for a time yet. Nearly three months later the mother wrote reporting a great improvement. The family home was some thirty miles from the clinic and she was so satisfied that she felt it unnecessary to return. Two years and two months after we first saw him she wrote: 'Lionel has improved tremendously, bad nights are a thing of the past, he eats well and is affectionate and friendly. He mutters that he'll chop me up one day with such venom that I almost believe it, and then smiles and says he didn't mean it!' The contrasting qualities of anger (resentment) and love, both directed towards his mother almost simultaneously, which the child's remarks reveal, are characteristic of the inner conflict which inevitably takes place in the mind of the child.

A girl was brought to the clinic at the age of one year and nine months, the younger daughter of a couple whom the therapist regarded as sound parents who had provided for their children a happy home, the problem being that she would not sleep at night, but lay awake, screaming. She had been a rhesus baby and required a complete transfusion at birth. Her mother was in good health during the pregnancy and confinement, but was not allowed to see her until she was forty-eight hours old, a circumstance which caused the mother great anxiety and which may have partially incapacitated her ability to handle the feeding problem which developed at once. For five days the baby was artificially fed and thereafter she would not feed at the breast, but by the time she came to the clinic she would take anything from a cup except milk, which she had from a bottle.

She seemed never to have been able to enjoy the suckling relationship and was therefore weaned at four months. She never was a cuddly baby, she walked at fifteen months and began to say single words at just over a year old. From the time of her weaning there seems to have been little further trouble until the age of sixteen months, but at that point she developed rages if not given whatever she wanted, and if picked up to stop her, she would bite. She knocked her sister about and pulled her hair. After four months the rages ceased (six weeks before she came to the clinic), but one night she woke at ten o'clock, screaming, and she continued to wake at ten or eleven every night and to scream till about four in the morning. At the same time she began to refuse to stay in her pram outside a shop, nor would she walk inside with her mother, but banged her head and had to be carried. She appeared an insecure, unsatisfied, unhappy child. It was relevant that her mother told us that she herself did not cry when she felt upset, but screamed and raised her voice, a matter on which her husband had commented to her.

The treatment was immediately a sedative at night for the child and also for her mother. We saw her father, too, an efficient, conscientious man, who told us that his wife was extremely uncomplaining and that she had one or two fads, one being that a dummy revolted her. We saw the mother in one or two further, counselling interviews and within six weeks she was able to report a satisfactory situation.

We saw the child again at the age of three years and a month. Her mother said that for a time she had had a habit of screaming if upset, but that she now had eczema instead. The sequence was usually a few days of poor sleep and of being rather unhappy, then two or three weeks of eczema but happy and well in other ways, and then a few days with no trouble at all before the cycle would begin again. But mother said she was managing to cope well with the situation. At this interview a large patch of eczema was visible on one thigh. Two years and two months after this interview the social worker paid a visit to the home and later remarked that the mother looked much happier than she used to be. The child, now more than five years of age, was attending school, where she had settled well, but she had become jealous of her older sister since starting school. Tantrums were less severe, but when she did have one her eczema would break out. She still had difficulty in getting to sleep, but once she was asleep she slept well till morning.

In support of a psychological etiology for these symptoms the disturbance caused by the transfusion and the deprivation occasioned by the two days' separation from her mother were likely to be of significance to the child, while the anxiety occasioned to her mother by these circumstances could also be influential. Yet these factors were hardly adequate as a full explanation of the problem, although the rapid improvement after she came to the clinic seemed to be in support of the psychological view as to causation. When, however, the eczema developed and revealed itself as a substitute for the screaming attacks which had preceded it, we had firmer grounds on which to build a theory of adverse constitutional loading as being an important and perhaps major factor in etiology. Our eventual diagnosis, therefore, was of an impaired capacity to adjust to the demands of the environment, accompanied by the abnormal rhesus factor and by the tendency to eczema, and due primarily to an anomaly of constitutional endowment. Such a view does not destroy the value of psychological treatment for the psychological difficulties with which both child and mother have to contend, but it provides a measure of comfort to those who have to handle the issues which are involved.

We have laid stress on the importance of trying to explain emotional illness on the basis of environmental influences, unless an organic basis is reasonably substantiated. It thus becomes almost a matter of policy in child guidance to seek the origins of the child's problem along avenues of emotion and cultural atmosphere. Perhaps we are helped in this by the viewpoint of the educational psychologist in the clinic who, coming from the teaching profession, is less likely than the doctor to be attracted by organic possibilities. At all events, the child having come to the clinic and having been examined and tested, it is our next objective to explain from the available evidence why the problem exists; and this exercise is to be undertaken purposefully, imaginatively even, at a stage when we still know too little to make for certainty.

We have found it an advantage to have a case summary in which the salient features are collected under specific headings and written in at the beginning of treatment, while further detail can be added later. Apart from its other uses this summary helps one to keep in mind the various factors pertaining to the case. The layout, a modification of one that used to be employed in the department of psychological medicine of University College Hospital, London, is given on the following page.

It can, of course, be adjusted so as to allow more room under headings likely to call for more space and the whole can conveniently be fitted on to one side of a piece of foolscap.

TREATMENT FOR CHILDREN

Case Summary

NAME   DATE OF BIRTH
ADDRESS   DATE OF FIRST INTERVIEW

REFERRED BY
FAMILY DOCTOR   SCHOOL

Problem and Related Symptoms:
Significant Points in Child's History:
Present Environment and Family History:
Intelligence and School Progress:
Type of Personality and Nature of Nuclear Problem:
Etiology of Problem:
Treatment Plans and Prospects:
Further Comments from Case Sheet:

CHAPTER II

Environmental Factors in Diagnosis and in Treatment

The Depth of the Problem
'The workers will have to assess whether the child's problems have become psychically internalized and so have come to have an independent existence apart from his surroundings, or whether the symptoms are a direct result of present-day environmental stress and would consequently be very much improved by direct modification of the child's surroundings and the forces which impinge upon him.'[4] We want to learn how the child evaluates the situation in which he lives. In those cases where the problem is internalized, where a true neurosis exists that is to say, it will usually be necessary to undertake treatment in the form of play therapy (psychotherapy) and this to be satisfactory may have to be lengthy. Even so, children have great powers of resilience and of recovery and if the child can achieve some understanding of his difficulty and a measure of increased self-confidence, and the parent a modicum of insight too, then a satisfactory level of improvement may be attained to in a relatively short space of time. If the problem is a more superficial reaction to circumstances, if the necessary adjustments can be made, whether at home, at school or elsewhere, and if the child sees that people are taking his difficulties seriously and are trying to help, the difficulty can sometimes be solved quite quickly. Given this background, even one or two psychotherapeutic interviews may enable the child to get the situation better into perspective, but we often have felt that it is the *interest* that people, especially his family, are showing in him that does most of the good work.

Human life being what it is in this industrial age, cases do not quite divide themselves into these two groups of the truly neurotic and the more superficial, types of problem. In the average child guidance clinic a big proportion of the work deals with the problems of children who, with their families have been caught up in the maze of industrialization and the acres of bricks and mortar that have ousted the countryside, and in the rat-race of materialism and the need to keep up with the Joneses. Whatever the term 'working class' may have implied in an earlier generation, it is now only too applicable, but in an altered sense, to many of our families today. It is under these circumstances that we find many of the children referred to our clinics to be the victims of what is, ultimately, a form of emotional rejection.

The drive for possessions, notably the motor car and the television set, and the way of life which such acquisitions represent has taken hold of people's minds. Mother goes out to work, father is preoccupied with aims and cares of his own, and when the children make demands there is a tendency to satisfy these with material gifts when what the children really need is the gift of their parents' time. It takes time to devote our love and our interest to our children and it is this kind of unselfishness which too often is lacking in the average modern family. Yet such neglect is neither purposeful nor deliberate, although it is the great modern sin of 'omission' and it is committed unawares. Child psychiatrists do well to be understanding but non-judgmental and we are reminded of a saying of Kenneth Cameron that 99 per cent of parents do their utmost for their children. Our task here is to help parents better to understand themselves.

Freud has said '. . . one may reasonably expect that . . . the conscience of the community will awake and admonish it that the poor man has just as much right to help for his mind . . . and the task will then arise for us to adapt our techniques to the new conditions. I have no doubt that the validity of our assumptions will impress the uneducated too, but we shall need to find the simplest and most natural expressions for our theoretical doctrines. . . . Possibly we may often be able to achieve something if we combine aid to the mind with material support.'[5]

The Child in the Family
In child guidance the superlatively important consideration is to realize the constant significance of interplay between the child and his parents, and to a less extent other members of the family. The apparent exception to this, the child who has been deprived of his family, will have been affected by his past neglect and will be continually under influence from the new family group or institutional community in which he is living. Soddy has made a basic contribution to our grasp of the meaning of the family in relation to problems which occur in children.[6]

The influence of environment is quite different, where the child is concerned, from what it is to the adult. The adult is a victim of that part of the ill in his past environment which lives on within his unconscious, and neurosis can be dealt with radically only by bringing these past influences, or their feeling content, into consciousness, where their effect on character can be rehashed. The child, by contrast, is actually in process of being influenced by present circumstances, and if their adverse qualities can be substituted by others which are more healthy, he may overcome his symptoms on a basis to some extent at least, of present reality. A baby we regard as being an integral part of his mother and she as being an incomplete unit without him. The young child's treatment, more often than not therefore, is to be done through her. Even the older child – to a diminishing degree once the teen years are reached – reacts so completely to the influences of his home that we must be constantly sensitive to parental attitudes *as a part of* whatever therapy the child receives. Sometimes in my own experience it has been necessary to treat a child without simultaneous contact with his mother, either because of a shortage of social workers or else because of the mother's poverty of co-operation, and again and again in these cases the lesson has been forced on us that if we are to get good results this defect must be repaired by bringing the mother into the orbit of the clinic's relationship with her child.

There are two aspects of this. The first is a simple one. Children are seldom ready to tell the therapist about their delinquencies, their disturbed behaviour or their fears, but tend to gloss over these and to give the impression that there has been greater amelioration of the problem than actually is the case. Unless information is available from home, usually through the social worker's contact with the mother, one is apt to be working in the dark or to believe that more success has attended the therapy to date than is actually the case. It is by no means appropriate that the therapist should usually tell the child that he has this information; the knowledge can be used in our conduct of the therapy without revealing our awareness of it. Sometimes I say: 'You will remember when you first came that Mummy said so-and-so. I wonder if this isn't perhaps still happening a good deal?' Occasionally I find it necessary to tell the child that I have heard something from Mummy – the child usually knows that she sees the social worker – and that I think we should talk about it.

The other aspect of this contact with the mother is a deeper one. Because the child is so dependent upon the influences in his home it often becomes necessary to effect changes in these influences if he is to have a fair chance of recovery. His mother's attitudes towards him and towards his symptoms – his anxieties, frustrations, resentments or demandingness – need explanation to her, while the wider relationships such as those between mother and father, may call for counselling.

Next usually in importance after mother herself is father. He often is less accessible, either because he cannot come to the clinic in working hours or because he refuses to come at all, and opportunities have been missed through not seeing a father. We ought to try to do this, and it is as well if the therapist himself can see the father, even if it means arranging an evening visit. An unwilling father, even if visited at home, may still be unwilling to contribute anything of his real feelings. Of course, one would not visit a father who has declined to accept such a visit. An improvement in family relationships is usually one of the major objectives in child guidance.

Sometimes a worker in one of our allied fields, probation officer or child care officer for example, is already in touch with the child's home. One of the faults of our social system is the manner in which the same family may find itself being visited by several different social workers all at the same time; but it is likely that the Government's plans for the integration of the social services will eventually eliminate this difficulty. At present we tend to ask the other worker, probation officer or whoever it is, to co-operate with the psychiatrist who is treating the child at the clinic, and the time of the social worker in the clinic is saved, to be available for someone else. This policy has generally worked well.

The social worker's rôle in treatment may fairly be described as complementary to that of the psychiatrist or therapist, a word that reminds us that neither is complete without the other. It has often been written that for the psychiatrist to be seeing the mother as well as the child may give the latter the feeling that the psychiatrist does not really belong to him or that he is not one in whom he can confide, because he is in league with parental authority. The more analytical the therapy the more likely is this to be the case and it is understandable that a child may be reluctant to express intimate feelings about his parents to someone who is in direct contact with them. He may also feel 'left out' by the psychiatrist's exclusion of him for a time, in order to see his mother. This could to a considerable extent be overcome by the psychiatrist seeing the mother at another time or by using the telephone. It is partly for the above reasons and partly because of the saving of the psychiatrist's time that we so widely adopt the system of therapist with child and social worker with mother. Generally speaking, however, in child guidance work one need not overrate the disadvantages of meetings between therapist and mother. On those occasions, and there have been many, where I have had to work without the help of a social worker, I have sometimes found it slightly awkward at the end of my interview with the child to be approached by his mother, who has asked how he is getting on, or has requested an interview. It is then better, if the question cannot be dealt with almost in a one-sentence answer, to say to the child that perhaps Mummy and I should have a little talk. Often, in fact, children are happy enough that the doctor should talk to mother. Nevertheless, the amount of time mothers need is often such as would cripple the psychiatrist's ability to get on with treatment, and there is thus a range of help which the social worker can provide, which would be beyond the therapist's capacity to undertake.

The social worker aims to make the child's mother feel that she herself is welcome at the clinic and that her co-operation is a part of therapy. There is a risk inherent in the psychological treatment of children that mothers may feel that they are being left out or that something is being done to their children which is outside their control. The social worker's enlistment of the mother's co-operation brings her right into the treatment circle. These factors are likely to be all the more important in the 'working-class' environment in which, more often than not, the clinic is situated.

When a grammar-school boy, approaching the age of thirteen, was referred for stealing, we decided at our clinic conference that he might be treated in a group which the psychiatrist was planning to run and that his mother should have help from the social worker. We felt that Charles[7] was in some degree a depressed child who felt unwanted, but at the end of three months the psychiatrist decided to let him stop coming to the group, partly because to do so involved him in missing important lessons at school. The satisfactory progress which he eventually achieved we regarded as mainly due to the social work, of which the social worker gave the following account.

I first became involved with this family when Charles came to the clinic, and I had regular contact with father and mother, together and separately, for almost two and a half years and have visited occasionally since.

Father was a tall, physically attractive man, who nevertheless had an outsize feeling of inferiority. This was possibly due to the fact that he was a member of a large family, all of whom received primary education on the pre-1944 plan, except the eldest boy, who won a scholarship to a grammar school, and about whom father said bitterly: 'Nothing was too good for him. He had everything, new clothes, uniform, cricket flannels, the lot, but we had anybody's left-offs.' This feeling was reinforced by Mrs Brackenhurst's attitudes. She disparaged her husband's abilities, despised his job as a barman and tended to suggest that Charles was of superior clay because he had passed the Eleven + and was in the local grammar school. Father felt himself unloved and had been jealous of Charles as a tiny baby – mother had somehow excluded him from contact with his baby son – and this jealousy had persisted, although he was now not so openly antagonistic to him.

Mother was a very anxious woman, overpossessive of her son, and inclined to turn for emotional satisfaction to him rather than to her husband. Prior to her marriage she had done some nursing training and was a state-enrolled assistant nurse. Her health was not good, she suffered from chronic nephritis and both her pregnancies had been difficult. Charles was the first child and she had spent most of this pregnancy in bed. Three years later they had another child, a girl who died after nine days, due it was said to a congenital heart lesion.

As I learned more about the ramifications of the family structure the picture became clearer and, as my relationship with them strengthened I tried to interpret Mr Brackenhurst to Mrs Brackenhurst and Charles's needs to both of them. Over the two and a half years of active social work with them my energies were directed towards changing Mrs Brackenhurst's attitude towards her husband and Mr Brackenhurst's attitude towards Charles and, as they were anxious to co-operate, their insight grew with each interview. Mr Brackenhurst no doubt unconsciously identified Charles with his eldest brother, and he transferred to his son all the emotions and conflicts which he had felt for his brother in his own childhood, and Mrs Brackenhurst had used Charles to punish her husband for unsatisfactory love relationships.

By the end of the period Mr Brackenhurst had changed his job to one which did not take him away from his family each night, his wife was doing clerical work on two afternoons a week and Charles had settled at school. He was doing better academically and was excelling at games. The whole family were happy and this situation has been maintained throughout the five years which have elapsed since regular counselling ceased. Charles, after leaving school, entered the field of professional athletics and his prospects appear reasonable.

Valuable to the therapist is the information which the social worker derives and which she can pass on to the therapist. To a smaller extent the social worker may give to the child's mother an idea of the kind of progress the therapy is making and also relieve the temptation the mother feels to question her child as to the content of the therapeutic interviews. It goes without saying that it is desirable she should ask her child no questions about his therapy, although she will be ready to listen to anything he wishes to say about it.

The social worker's next task is that of understanding the child's mother herself in order that she may counsel her in her handling of her child. Mothers often are under pressure to criticize, to make demands on behaviour, to scold or to punish, or else they worry about the child's symptoms, feel themselves guilty about his problems or compare him unfavourably with other children. Direct advice could easily defeat its own object by creating further anxiety in a mother who already is the victim of her own emotional drives, but if the social worker *understands* the child's mother she will be able to give her counselling the sort of twist which will transform it into an experiment in child handling, which mother, social worker and father can all share.

Punishment is a topic that is bound to come up in our discussions with mothers. In contemplating the punishment of a child parents could usefully be made aware of the fact that the urge to punish arises from the adult's own unconscious resentments against authority figures of his childhood for whose sins his own child is now going to be made to pay the penalty. Mother's smack applied in the heat of the moment may be less harmful than the delayed thrashing inflicted after a period of time. Yet during this time the parent might have reflected upon what were his child's needs rather than being swayed by what were his own, or society's, retributive impulses. Isaacs[8] has clearly shown that a child's own inner feeling of guilt is normally much stronger than any that will arise from punishment inflicted externally, so that the whole case usually made out for punishment as being guilt provoking, and therefore potentially remedial, simply falls away. So often it is the parent who becomes upset, because the child's 'naughtiness' activates the parent's own complex-motivated anxieties and guilt feelings, who responds angrily or punitively. With those parents who are intelligent and are not completely dominated by their own emotions I try to explain the operation of these mental mechanisms, in the hope that the parent will be able to accept the child's foibles more dispassionately, rather than by becoming upset by them, and thus will be able to react towards the child purposefully rather than impulsively.

One situation which deserves mention is that of the child who is behaving fretfully or naughtily and who feels so guilty about it that he needs to be punished in order to relieve these feelings. This state of affairs is one circumstance under which appropriate punishment at the time can be relieving to the child's feelings and thus beneficial.

Inevitably the mother's own problems and her unconscious drives will focus themselves upon the social worker's attention and those mothers who are themselves neurotic will present special difficulties. To counsel them with any sort of adequacy will be tantamount to taking the mother on for treatment. Psychiatric social workers do, of course, treat patients, as witness the excellent work of the Institute of

Marital Studies.[9] It is a good rule in child guidance that whenever possible the social worker should keep her interviews with the mother at the level of counselling in matters of handling the child, of the meaning of the child's problem and of parental attitudes towards him. If it clearly becomes necessary to go beyond this and to deal specifically with the mother's own inner difficulties, then the question will have to be decided as to whether the social worker should undertake this or whether the mother should be referred to another psychiatrist. This will depend upon a number of local considerations of which not the least will be the social worker's own skill, aptitudes and inclinations.

Treatment Necessary for the Mother.
Now and again it will turn out that once the whole situation of the child in his family has been assessed the policy that seems most profitable is that the mother should have psychiatric treatment. Because of the pressure of work on surrounding adult psychiatric clinics and the general shortage of psychotherapists, this is not always easy to arrange, and it may be necessary for the child psychiatrist to undertake this therapy if it is to be done at all. Occasionally this is the proper course. It will mean that the child is not taken on for treatment, but, in the cases of younger children at least, if the mother is given adequate help this may well suffice.

Administrative considerations should be taken seriously. The family doctor, school medical officer, teacher or whoever has referred the child to the clinic has an indirect but none the less real part in therapy. The important thing here is communication and this rests on a basis of trustful understanding between the person who refers the child and the staff of the clinic. Given this element of mutual regard, it matters little whether the communication is by letter, telephone or personal visit. What is harmful is want of this sympathetic regard for each other, because that can result in working at cross-purposes, a circumstance which is likely to lay an added emotional strain on the child and which is obviously unfair to him.

Child guidance, unlike medicine or surgery in hospital, calls for a system of constant and healthy co-operation between workers whose professional skills stem from varied disciplines. The psychiatrist and the social worker have their roots in a medically fertilized soil, while the psychologist, and perhaps the clinic secretary who is also an important member of the staff, will have many of their ideas stemming from the educational field. By no means all the doctors with whom the clinic has to co-operate share all the clinic's attitudes, while teachers, whose acceptance of our work can be quite vital, vary widely in their

THE ENVIRONMENT

approach. Other allies of the clinic are those who live in a more legal milieu, notably probation and child care officers, although it often is they who, more than most, think along the same lines as ourselves.

It cannot be otherwise than that many of those workers will differ from us in one or another point of view, varying from frank suspicion to mere differences in detail, and jealousies there must be. The child psychiatrist has, therefore, to be someone who can accept these differences and can assimilate them into his ways of thinking and working. After all, the 'difficult' colleague is a colleague who has problems, and if we can think of him, or of her, in this way we may find ourselves becoming more tolerant. The psychiatrist who becomes exasperated about a situation is one who has emotional problems of his own, and in such an event self-examination may be the remedy.

A boy came to our clinic within weeks of the date for his leaving school finally. He had come to our area from another place, with a history of long treatment for school phobia, which had included excusal from school attendance. We were told that his attendance since he had come to our town had been negligible, and the psychiatrist's inclination had been to write a certificate excusing him on medical grounds for the remainder of the present final term and to offer treatment appointments. He was the sort of boy who presented the bland exterior of the hysteric and who felt quite justified in saying that as he could not bring himself to go to school he had the right not to go.

In our subsequent discussion the psychologist considered it unwise that we should encourage so easy a way out to someone who was, after all, evading a legal obligation to attend school. We therefore decided that the psychiatrist would collect the boy at his home, take him to school and discuss with him and the headmaster what adjustments might be made in the school programme in order to accommodate the boy's difficulties. The headmaster was most co-operative; the psychiatrist and the boy saw him in school together and a suitable plan was worked out. The boy failed to honour his part of the bargain and did not return to school any more, nor did he come back to the clinic. The record may be interesting if he turns up later at an adult clinic. Within the clinic the experience strengthened our working relationship.

A girl in her last year at school had recently come with her family from another town and because of fainting attacks both the hospital and our own clinic had investigated carefully. Our social worker's visit to the home, and especially the father's attitude there, had been difficult; drug therapy had been commenced, on account of a neurological consideration, and we had decided to see her in regular interviews for a time. One day she came to tell us that her father refused to allow her to see us any more. A passive handling of this situation seemed necessary. The position had to be accepted and when we had made sure that the girl was not so unhappy at home as actually to wish to leave home we made it clear that we should welcome a visit if ever she wished to come back. Subsequently she came under the care of the probation officer and we were able to be in touch once more.

Our cordial relationships with the children's department are occasionally ruffled by what seems a too possessive or bureaucratic attitude on their part. One of their girls, who was with good foster-parents, had been behaving in such a way at school that the children's department and the headmistress asked us to do something about it, and we arranged her admission to a special hospital. This had been months ago; the girl was still in the hospital, and what we were now told was that her foster-mother was confused about arrangements for her to come home at Eastertime. We were told that some time back the physician at the hospital had written to the foster-mother and had been thereafter asked by the children's department, who were the legal guardians, not to do so. We decided to ignore this up to a point and we got round the difficulty by addressing the letter to the children's officer, but sending copies to the foster-mother and to anyone else directly concerned, in order to be sure that the Easter holiday arrangements were satisfactory.

The headmaster of a boy with whom we had been in close touch had, in our view, been guilty of handling him unfairly, and to make matters a little worse, we knew that he had told the principal school medical officer that he was quite unaware that we were dealing with the boy, a statement which the psychologist, who had visited him at school, could not credit as having been made honestly. The headmaster had, in fact, rebuffed the educational psychologist on the occasion of her visit, but she recognized that he himself was under some emotional strain of which his treatment of the boy was in some way a symptom. She decided to handle the affair by tactful telephone conversations as a preliminary to the effecting of whatever changes were going to be in the boy's interest.

A boy, well known to the clinic and to whom we were giving a good deal of active help at the time, was before the magistrates for one of the relatively harmless peccadilloes in which he was in the habit of indulging. The psychiatrist, after invitation to do so, submitted a carefully considered report to the Court. The magistrates' response was to say they wanted more information, to send the boy to a remand home – he had just had nine days in camp with us and the justices knew that – and to have it arranged that another psych-

THE ENVIRONMENT

iatrist, who knew nothing of him or of his past, would see him. Nor was this the first instance of its kind and there had been occasions when subsequent events had proved the clinic's recommendations to be right. On the present occasion the psychiatrist mentioned to the medical officer of health his disappointment with the Court's attitude and with the justices' ignorance of the meaning of our work, with the result that an arrangement was made for the psychiatrist to address a meeting of magistrates.

In the case of a dull and emotionally unstable boy who had been referred to the clinic we had, after careful investigation, recommended that he should go to the residential school for educationally subnormal children, to have this overruled by the authorities. Within a year or so the boy was before the magistrates on a charge. On another occasion we made the strongest possible appeal that a boy with whom we had had considerable dealings should have a place at a residential school for maladjusted children. Although usually they were cooperative, in this particular instance the Education Department absolutely refused. In course of time the High Court sentenced the boy to a long term of imprisonment for behaviour which not unlikely would have been avoided had our request been granted.

What does one do about these things? They can be personally distressing, neither annoyance nor argument is likely to be of avail, and persuasion sometimes fails. Realizing how inevitable it is that other folk will sometimes dig their heels in, in a view that is contrary to our own, it is often best simply to accept these arbitrary decisions as being unavoidable in this imperfect world. What, however, has been a measure of great value in many cases where there has been a difference of opinion has been to invite the other person to meet the child psychiatrist in discussion, and it has often been found that if the psychiatrist's time is precious, the colleague will be willing to come over to the clinic. A great deal, though not everything, can be ironed out in this way.

Still another kind of case is that where a parent is aggrieved by the attitude of some authority, education for example. What matters is not which point of view the psychiatrist favours but the fact that he is by his training and by the central position which he occupies, in a better position than anybody else to interpret one side to the other and to allay the anxieties of the parents, of the child, or of the caseworker who is involved from the 'official' side. In all this the writer sometimes sees himself as being the possessor of the oil-can, judicious application of the contents of which can calm many troubled stretches of water.

Stresses within the clinic can be more damaging than those without and it is bound to happen that there will be cases where the personalities of members of a clinic team will clash with each other. If this happens, short of one or other worker actually leaving the clinic, some remedy must be found, and it is unlikely that one of the professional workers will accept treatment, which would possibly be the best answer. Two guiding lines I have found to be of real merit in dealing with such difficulties. The first is that, just as the psychiatrist is accustomed to regard the child's personality as being one part of a problem that calls for understanding and patient handling and the mother's personality as being a second, similar part, so he should mentally treat the colleague who is not easy to get along with as presenting a part of the problem, so that one comes to make almost the same kind of allowance for the colleague's awkwardness as one does in the case of child or parent. If this is done with humble sincerity it can work. The second guiding line is a preparedness on the part of the psychiatrist to defer to the wishes of another member of the team who has strong views on some issue. It is occasionally useful to remind oneself that the purpose of the work we are doing together is to make the lives of children happier, and if the co-operation between the members of the team which fosters this purpose can be advanced by the psychiatrist's willingness to yield, the gains may outweigh the losses. How far one is prepared to carry this must be a matter for idiosyncratic decision and especially in any case where a child's interests might be harmed the psychiatrist must, in discussion, state his opinions quite clearly.

The *maximum age* at which a girl or boy will be accepted by a child guidance clinic is in many cases geared for administrative convenience to the age when he leaves school, so that as the school-leaving age rises so does the age for acceptance at the clinic. Medically it is not easy to defend such a policy and a better criterion would appear to be whether or not the young person is sufficiently adult to benefit from the kind of treatment available in the adult psychiatric clinic. Psychiatrists working in the adult field are not always familiar with the best methods of approach to the inhibited middle teenager and there is much to be said for allowing anyone up to the age of seventeen to come to the child guidance clinic.

CHAPTER III

The Unconscious Origin of Neurosis

Time and again, where the origin of a nervous problem has been in doubt, the real explanation has turned out to be a sexual one. An example of this arose in the case of a boy who was referred to us at the age of twelve and a half, the complaint being that he had suffered from psychosomatic pains ever since he commenced school at the age of five, and that he was unhappy, was friendless and had been stealing. His I.Q. was 110, but he was bottom of the class, he cried at night over his homework, he did not like school and he was teased by other boys. His mother was a warm personality, but his father had a bitter streak in his make-up and the couple were not happy with each other.

In the clinic the therapist came to have a good relationship with the boy, who attended, with intermissions which were by the therapist's arrangement, for a period of well over a year. In the summer he came to camp with us in two successive years. In therapy many matters were explored and some, if not all, of the symptoms improved to varying degrees. Yet he remained basically maladjusted within his environment, a shut-in personality. Why, one wondered, had this boy not been brought to see us at the age of five? The therapist became convinced that there was some problem within the boy's conscious awareness, but which he would not reveal. How one becomes thus convinced is not easy to explain – it is a sort of hunch, the weighing together of various factors and the experience learned in earlier cases that some children knew more than they would tell. Various specific possibilities were explored – masturbation, the possibility that he felt he was different from other boys, and the therapist even wondered if the boy thought he was, or might become, mentally abnormal – but when brought up in interview none yielded a positive result.

At the end of twenty interviews this shut-in, ungiving attitude persisted, and the therapist was talking of masturbation anxieties, concern over girls, father's want of understanding and whatever else seemed relevant, but without obtaining any response. In the following interview the boy painted a country scene with two symmetrical hillocks, a river flowing between them down to the fields below, a bridge, three rabbits, a tree and many birds. The hillocks and the river could have represented breasts and milk, but the selected interpretation was of a wish to withdraw into a paradise of responsibility-free childhood. It was at this point that the therapist concluded that there was some problem which was being consciously concealed. He went over the issues again with him, referred once more to his inability to trust the therapist and said that he felt it would be best to discontinue the interviews, but that the boy could come back to him if ever he wanted his help later on.

This boy went home and told his mother what the therapist had said, and added: 'Why should I tell him? I want to keep it to myself.' The therapist saw the mother at this juncture. Reflecting on the case, he concluded that there were two possibilities. The first was that the boy might fear some sexual damage, although this was something that had been covered pretty thoroughly during the interviews. The other possibility was that the boy might be afraid of going mad. When this was mentioned to his mother she said that her son had once said to his big brother: 'It's because I'm going off the deep end.' Soon after this, however, he did tell his mother that his concern arose from the fact that he was the only boy in his school class who had been circumcised and that his penis looked feeble compared with those of his mates.

This could not be the inner source of his anxieties, but it was their focal point. The boy returned and in three further interviews the therapist was able to deal reassuringly with his doubts. This appeared to be all that was necessary. Looking back afterwards at the last painting, with this knowledge, one was struck by the likeness to a lithotomy view, with the little hills as testicles and the stream as the urinary flow. The birds in the painting could have possible relevance in that in current adolescent terminology the word 'bird' was widely used to mean 'girl'. During a period of several months about this time this boy suffered from a form of spinal osteitis; he left school shortly afterwards at the age of fifteen and it is to his credit that, in spite of the nature of this recent disability, he was accepted for boy service in the Navy. He has done well since.

As we shall see shortly, these present anxieties are likely to have received their forcefulness from much earlier and more fundamental fears. The influence of stress, producing emotions, on the plastic mind of the infant, is immeasurably stronger than the effects of later experiences can be on the partially formed mentality of the school child.

The Growth of Understanding

It will be worth while to consider how the baby's understanding grows and to examine the phases of development through which psychoanalytical study has shown that children pass.[10] There is no certain evidence that the newborn baby possesses consciousness or that birth trauma has any psychological effect, despite some emotional material that is suggestive of the latter. In any case, the child is almost continuously asleep. The consciousness of the early months of life is quite different from what we understand as the consciousness of adults. It is not an intellectual appreciation but a kind of awareness or feeling. The baby experiences feeling, intensely in fact, but there is no intellectual understanding or verbalization, for the comprehension of meanings and words is as yet in the remote future.

In the early weeks *intellectual appreciation* dawns. At first there is a vague awareness of mother. This becomes more defined and is followed by awareness of objects and of other persons. Along with this development comes an awareness of his own body and an inclination to explore both himself and objects in the world outside.

In the psychomotor field the pyramidal tracts are still unmyelinated at birth and the baby has no power of neuromuscular co-ordination. Only crying and alimentary and urinary mechanisms are organized. About 75 per cent of babies are deaf at birth and there is little sound perception for fourteen days; 50 per cent will close their eyes to moderate light, and after a month the baby will fix a light with his eyes. The skin is relatively insensitive for some weeks and taste discrimination is poor up to about nine months. Sensitivity to bowel tension appears very early in life.

At birth the grasp reflex is present, a startle reflex by the second week and at eight weeks head-raising when lying prone. A reflex smile may occur before the age of three months, and the social smile, directed to his mother (and later on to others) appears at four to six months. At four months the baby will follow an object with his eyes. At four or five months he will raise his head from the supine position. He may recognize persons from about six months onward. An average child will probably sit up, unsupported, at eight months and will walk at eleven to sixteen months, most usually about fourteen months. Talking may be expected to begin early in the second year. Some children will feed themselves with a spoon at one year. In the first half of the second year exploring the environment is the child's chief interest; from six months to twelve or eighteen months there is much exploratory behaviour, picking up toys and setting them down, but without, as yet, any idea of the significance of toys.

The oral phase of emotional gratification extends from birth to about the end of the first year. Instinctively the baby *sucks* and he enjoys this experience. *Frustration in relation to feeding* is almost the earliest cause of anxiety. The baby who must wait unduly or who is unsatisfied at the end of his feeds, and whose inherent capacity to tolerate frustration is less than average, will develop a rage reaction and this may be coupled with fear. This may be reflected in later life by inability to bear opposition of any kind.

It is important that a mother should not only feed her baby but, almost equally so, that she should love and cuddle him. The experience of being caressed, of being loved, is a requirement without which a baby cannot thrive. Furthermore, if the child does not experience being loved and being able to reciprocate love, he will never be able later on to acquire the capacity to make healthy love relationships in the family or in society. The now famous work of Bowlby and his colleagues has shown that there is a close relationship between love deprivation and the development of psychopathic personality. Breast feeding *as such* is not the important thing: bottle feeding is comparably good if the love relationship is there. Even so, the present-day decline in breast feeding is a matter for regret.

Rejection, whether at this early stage of life or later on, is frequently the origin of nervous breakdown. Some children are rejected by their mothers. This may be simply because the mother does not want her child, or it may arise from less conscious factors such as immaturity and the emotional need to be a child herself. Some mothers are themselves cold (psychopathic?) and cannot be loving. Occasionally a child such as the fourth in a working-class family may be very neglected about the age of two or three years, and 'good', quiet babies of over-pressed mothers tend to be neglected. The sense of insecurity thus engendered is a fertile cause of neurotic anxiety, and sometimes of aggression and delinquency later. Two cardinal signs of disturbance in mother-child symbiosis are *gastro-enteritis* and *bronchitis*.

The late Dr Hardcastle had a patient in psychoanalysis who suddenly said, just out of the blue and with considerable feeling: 'Why is it that mothers frustrate their babies so infuriatingly by not letting them get to the breast?' What had happened was that this man had, in his feelings during analysis, gone back to the early weeks of life; and these words now emerging were simply the expression of the fact that he at that moment felt himself a baby, longing to get milk from his mother's breast.

It is worth explaining that the patient in analysis does not *remember* such an occasion – the feeling, not the intellectual recollection, comes into consciousness. One of my own patients, when having psychotherapy from me in her twenties, found that when walking along the road she felt she was herself coming home from school. She did not imagine this, but felt it to be so and it frequently was difficult for her to come out of this existence into present-day reality.

Ideally a baby should not have to suffer a greater degree of frustration than he can contain or assimilate. If he does suffer more than he can handle he will become neurotic, which means that in later life he will react to the frustration with such symptoms as anxiety and anger. Thus the roots of neurotic reaction or the basis of mentally healthy reactions are laid down very early in life. Factors which later on appear to cause mental upset are activating, rather than genuinely causative, and only exceptionally will these later difficulties be sufficiently severe to cause neurosis in a person not already predisposed. This does not mean that treatment later on will be valueless. Analysis gives a patient insight into his primitive emotions and thus enables changes to take place. Children are still in the phase of development, they have great powers of recovery, and if factors which are activating a problem can be ameliorated the child may in measure overcome the problem even though it also has earlier roots. This helps to explain why, though a few children will need analysis if they are to recover, many more can be helped by the methods of child guidance treatment. Yet it is an advantage if the therapist is himself analytically orientated, so that he can grasp the existence of deeper causes as well as of more obvious influences. In many cases he will interpret present-day difficulties in terms of these unconscious mechanisms and will select parts of this interpretation to be passed on to the child whom he is treating, or sometimes to the parent.

One of the writer's adult patients said she wondered what parents meant when they said they loved their children, because everything had, as it were, to be bought by the children in the coin of conforming behaviour. Discussion led on to the fact that the patient had lately been eating a great deal between meals.

D.[11] Do you know what this means?

P. (*quoting her mother*) 'Jacqueline, don't gobble your food up' . . . Dad was always asking about food . . . My parents were always short of food.

D. Were you short of food when you were very small?

P. I don't know: I was kept short of love.

D. Do you think that food and love might be the same thing?

P. Perhaps. Mother made so much of food.

D. There's one other connection you have not yet got . . . the situation at the breast.

P. Mother did starve me, I am told, and I didn't gain. They had to put me on the bottle . . . That's queer . . . odd . . . it seems to

link up with it . . . she commenced to suck her finger quite audibly . . . and I'm sucking my finger!
D. So that is what is happening when you eat voraciously now.
P. Being denied the essentials of life.
D. Love. The giving of food represents love.

A boy of nine came to see us on the recommendation of the speech therapist who had been treating him for multiple dyslalia in which there had been appreciable improvement. He also wet his bed, he had temper tantrums, was afraid of the dark, had stolen and was very possessive of mother. His I.Q. was 78, an earlier assessment having been slightly less than this, and he was the second of four children in a happy family, although there had been some domestic difficulties in the early years of the marriage. Towards his younger sister he displayed considerable antipathy. His mother had had some gynaecological trouble and had suffered from depressive symptoms, but it was the social worker's opinion that she had always been rejecting of Benjamin. For four years he had been known both to the speech therapist and to our social worker, but only now, it seemed, was he considered to need serious child guidance attention. The psychiatrist assessed him as being a generally insecure child of below average intelligence and he felt that special regard should be paid to the aggression which was undoubtedly related to this insecurity. We decided to take Benjamin for a short series of treatment sessions.

In the first of these sessions he painted a duck attacking a boat and the therapist interpreted the boat as his mother, father and the home situation, which he, the duck, was attacking because he felt they were not being good to him. He was prepared passively to accept this, but a subsequent attempt on the therapist's part to get Benjamin to tell him something of his school difficulties met with no response and the therapist realized that Benjamin could as yet trust him very little and that he, the therapist, would have to make the going.

In the third interview Benjamin painted a submarine striking at a boat which was raising anchor. The therapist led the discussion towards feelings of anger and Benjamin said that when the submarine got back home everyone on land was dead, as the submarine had blown up the land. The therapist said that this resembled the guilt we felt about our own anger and the badness in us. It must have been very frightening to the submarine to find how much harm it had done and so we felt sometimes that we might be punished for our anger. The therapist had, in fact, commenced this interview by saying something about anger and resultant guilt, but he had made no suggestion as to what kind of picture Benjamin might paint. In the next interview Benjamin looked pretty sad and tended to suck his thumb. He didn't accept a suggestion that he felt they did not love him at home, but he agreed that he felt they did not care very much. In the following session Benjamin said he still wet his bed and was angry at times. Arithmetic was giving him difficulty and the therapist wondered if the educational psychologist might be able to mollify his teacher's expectations.

In later interviews there was further talk about anger. Benjamin painted a pleasant picture of two cows in grassland. There were several 'pancakes' (faeces of cows) around and one of the cows was defecating, its dung actually falling through the air. The therapist felt that enough had been gained, that any further progress would be very slow and that it would be appropriate to stop, although keeping in touch for some time in the future. The speech therapist saw Benjamin once again and considered that his speech was potentially satisfactory. His mother said that he was appreciably better, although the jealousy situation continued to be in evidence.

At the end of the last interview, as his mother was standing in the passage with her arm across her chest, Benjamin played with her hand, biting it gently. The scene was impressively reminiscent of a calf suckling from the cow – a reminder that treatment should concern itself with elemental needs.

The anal phase of gratification succeeds the oral at about the age of a year and extends to about two and a half, although overlapping considerably with the oral phase and with the genital phase which follows on from it. In the anal phase the baby's 'feeling' interest is transferred somewhat from preoccupation with mouth sensations to those centred around the excretory functions. He tends to be more obstinate and not easily diverted and displays qualities of aggressiveness and demandingness. This level of development is sometimes called 'anal-sadistic' and elements of fixation to this level, when they reveal themselves in adult life, are characterized by sadistic tendencies. The child in this phase has no empathy of his mother's reactions – she is someone who is there only for his good – and the delightful quality of wanting to please his mother does not appear until a later stage. If his mother is too demanding herself at this time, he may refuse to co-operate. He shows ambivalence of feeling, one moment loving her and the next moment attacking. He has no concern for the rights of others and there is much rage reaction if he is frustrated. A group of two-year-old children cannot be left alone together or they would harm each other.

The baby at this time obtains satisfaction from defecation. The faeces have value for him. They are, after all, the only object he is able to produce and can be a gift. If mother does not show appreciation of the gift – e.g. if she shows disgust – it may be withheld (constipation). They may also be a weapon, and soiling a symptom of revenge for neglect, real or imagined, or for what the child feels to be want of love on his mother's part. In this way resort to soiling on the part of an already clean child may be his reaction to the hurt and jealousy he feels when a baby brother or sister is born. This is an example of *regression* to an earlier stage of life.

Too early or too strict *toilet training* may give rise to personality difficulties. Pre-trained children play with faeces. In this, and in soiling generally, the child comes up against his mother's refusal to condone the continuance of the habit. He may then overvalue the 'dirtiness' of his bowel contents and may become anxious, so that he may go excessively over to the side of the angels and become more deeply upset by his soiling than his mother is. This may result in a refusal of 'nasty' food like meat (which is coloured like faeces) or eggs. The effect of training has then been a *reaction-formation* which in some cases goes so far that the child becomes obsessional about cleanliness, there being a *displacement* of the emotion from the soiling to these foods. Reaction formation means that some forbidden or dangerous emotion has been repressed below consciousness and that there has grown up a strong feeling of repugnance against it at the conscious level. Another example relates to unconscious, infantile, incestuous desires, *vide infra*, which are represented in later life by strong, conscious repugnance against incest. Forbidden desires may thus be dealt with, in part at least, by the substitution of their opposites.

Guilt regarding forbidden wishes may cause them to be dealt with by *denial*. A little girl who has had desire for the boy's sexual organ may later deny that boys have a penis, or a child who has felt sexual desire and become guilty about it may deny the possibility that her parents have had sexual intercourse.

Projection means that we attribute to others the bad feeling in ourselves. A child who has 'done wrong' may attribute the naughty behaviour not to himself but to sister, brother or doll. We sometimes come across *splitting of the personality*, some children having good and bad names for the 'good' and 'bad' halves of themselves.

Fantasy life is an important part of childhood experience, a part of which consists in replacing painful realities with pleasurable imaginations.

The phallic, or genital phase of childhood extends from the age of around two and a half years to about six or seven, and is at its height at about the age of five. There is a preoccupation with the external genital organs, and exploratory touching and looking, as well as

UNCONSCIOUS INFLUENCES

pleasure in the sensation of touching, evolve as emotional outlets. This kind of play cannot fairly be called masturbation.[12] There are, nevertheless, a number of children who are given to gross indulgence in stroking or rubbing their sexual organs, which does seem to amount to masturbation; in these cases it will nearly always be found, if the home background is carefully explored, that there is some form of emotional deprivation and that the child's needs are being subordinated to those of his parents. Tender and loving feelings are characteristic of the phallic phase. Children make friendships at the age of four, manliness develops and the child wants to exhibit his achievements. Girls display maternal qualities.

The influence and importance of the parents' attitudes are paramount. If father is rough with mother the little boy may ape this attitude. Selfishness, quarrelsomeness or obstinacy on the part of one or both of his parents may cause the child to adopt similar attitudes, or recoiling from this behaviour he may go over to its opposite and support the parent who, he feels, is being injured, or he may repress his anxious or aggressive impulses and so develop an insecure, nervous personality. The inhibited, insecure child, unable adequately to exteriorize his feelings and desires, is, in my experience, perhaps the major problem facing child psychiatry in our industrialized society. The eventual impact of such development on adult mental health is too obvious to require emphasis.

The Oedipus complex arises during the genital phase because once the infant's libido[13] has progressed to a genital sexual level there emerge desires of libidinal gratification with the parent of the opposite sex. Up till now every pregenital desire has more or less been gratified by the parent: now for the first time the child comes up against a wall of total parental refusal to gratify these wishes.[14] This wish for gratification with his mother naturally produces a sense of rivalry towards his father, who is stealing his mother from him, and in his hatred of his father he may in fantasy destroy him. For the little girl the complex is similar, but she has a more difficult adjustment to make, because her mother, who was her first love, has been supplanted in her desires by her father. Even where a parent has died, the complex still operates in much the same way, as some other adult, whether in reality or in fantasy, takes the place of the absent parent.

Much of the evidence for all this is of a psychoanalytical nature, and those of us who have not been analysed find it difficult to conceive that we did ourselves actually have such incest wishes. Another of my adult patients could remember, before the age of three, being sexually aroused by his mother bathing him. Not only was he aroused by her handling him in this way, but she used sometimes, while he was in his bath, to pass water seated on the water closet which was in the same room. This made him very excited. Here was an openly sexual longing and the case presents for us a picture of what is in fact a universal experience. However much adult consciousness may dislike the idea, little children do have tremendously strong emotional desires in relation to the genital and anal orifices of their own bodies and those of others.

The term 'incestuous wish' has been used to describe these feelings, but by using this term we do not mean that the baby desires to have sexual intercourse with his parent in an adult orientation. The little child feels a tremendous, possessive love, a strong sensual desire, and this is channelled to the sex organs emotionally. Thus the little boy has an intense desire to *possess* his mother in the sensual, infantile-sexual manner which is the natural expression of feelings at that age. The little girl, similarly, entertains such feelings – feelings be it noted and not conceptualized thoughts – for her father.

An older patient of mine told me that her father had tried to have an incestuous relationship with her while bathing her as a little girl. She had certainly been very attached to him and had a good deal of unresolved resentment regarding his death, which had taken place in the meantime, but her mother assured me that it was impossible for this story of sexual misbehaviour on his part to be true. Freud, in his researches into this subject, was interested to find that a number of his patients told of such sexual assaults by their fathers, but he later discovered that these assaults had not actually taken place. His patients were not lying. They believed in the occurrences, but their beliefs were fantasies, and I am satisfied that, in the case of my own patient, this was also a fantasy. What is the origin of such fantasies? Freud was able to grasp their inner meaning, namely that the basis of such fantasies is desire, and that in expressing them as believed-in realities patients are really telling us of their intensely strong, unconscious wishes. It is easy to recognize that an adolescent will have strong emotional interest in the sexual organs of an attractive person of the opposite sex. What is important for us is to be able to grasp that the baby has an equally strong, though less differentiated, pleasure interest (libido) in the excretory and sexual orifices.

When the patient to whom I have referred was ten years of age her father was killed in an accident. But in her interviews with me she insisted that he had committed suicide. Of her mother she said: 'I hated mother before father was killed' – evidence of her intellectual knowledge of the actual circumstances of her father's death, though she 'knew' emotionally that he had deserted her by suicide. 'Mother was in the way. Sometimes I hate her just because she fed me.' The last sentence apparently indicates the existence of a complex of frustration going back to breast feeding, but the rest of the story betokens an unresolved Electra complex, the female counterpart of the Oedipus complex. In the fable Electra and her sister killed their mother in order to avenge the death of their father.

These sensual desires of infantile sex feeling are opposed by the experience of absolute parental disapproval or prohibition and this results in feelings of aggression against the parent who thus denies to the child expression of his libidinous wish. But this aggression leads on to a fear of reprisal for these aggressive feelings in the form of overwhelming punishment. In this lies the origin of much of the unconscious guilt which can lead to depression later in life.

A little girl was frolicking around the room in great glee. Her knickers, slipped down to her ankles, by restricting freedom of movement, gave just the necessary odd quality to the occasion, and as she tripped around, caressed her baby sister and basked in her grandmother's approval, she seemed in the seventh heaven of delight. All of a sudden she burst into tears – bitter, unconsolable, terrified tears. Asked what was wrong she just said: 'My Daddy says this is wicked'. For a full half-hour this uncontrollable pathos continued; nothing could comfort her and more than once the above statement was repeated. As it turned out, her father had said nothing that could ordinarily be expected to carry such a meaning and the only explanation was that this was his fantasied disapproval. Emotions carrying this degree of pain or terror can be handled by the child only by *repression*, by being forgotten that is, but it was as though for one half-hour the painful unconscious was laid open to the light of day.

The Oedipus complex is the crucial factor in human emotional development and on its satisfactory solution subsequent mental health will often depend. The solution involves repression of the libidinal wishes and it is this which, as we shall shortly see, ushers in the latency period.

Castration Anxieties. Even before the Oedipus stage of development the super-ego had had origins in any of the circumstances under which the mother has frustrated the child's libido in its oral or anal expression. The *super-ego* may be described as that part of the emotions which causes a person to feel self-blame or to be self-critical and which leads on to feelings of unworthiness or of guilt. Parental prohibition has been *introjected* and has become a force within the personality which forbids or limits libidinal expression. Introjection means that the child takes into his own mental life the attitudes, prohibitions, moral standards, cultural patterns or behavioural qualities of his parents, so that their attributes become his by being incorporated into his own personality, This force is the super-ego and it is now, in the genital phase of development, the parental non-co-operation with or frustration of the oedipal desires which gives to the super-ego its greatest access of strength. There develops in the child's fantasy a fear of *castration*, and this evidently combines fear of talion punishment in the form of the actual loss of the sexual organ, with at the same time an emotional castration in the form of destruction or repression of libidinal expression. One outcome of the failure to resolve this complex is the inhibition of expression which is so characteristic of many of the children we see in the child guidance clinic. Talion punishment is described by Berg as: 'Retaliatory punishment. Punishment equivalent to the crime. The principle of "eye for eye, tooth for tooth".'

The structure of fantasy on which a castration fear rests may be complicated, but a little boy who has seen that his sister has no penis may well wonder why. There have also been authenticated cases of direct threats made to a child that his penis will be cut off, usually as a punishment for masturbation. In this fear we may also see something of the origins of masturbation guilt. Where no actual threat has been made a fantasied threat nevertheless arises. A lady patient whom I treated a number of years ago told me that as a child she had been afraid to look at the genital part of her body. When asked, 'Afraid to look?' she replied: 'Because I'd lost something.' Asked how she had lost it, she quietly said: 'I feel as if it had been pulled off.' At the age of six she accidentally cut her head and was taken to hospital. She believed that her head was going to be cut off.

Although there is adequate evidence to prove the existence of a fantasy of mutilation of this kind, it may be easier to conceive of the emotion as being a fear of emasculation of a wider type, an emotional castration. If, that is to say, the oedipal castration fear complex has not been solved, the child feels different from others, afraid of life's relationships and unable to make strong, positive identifications with hero figures. The main plank of treatment will be the formation of a relationship with the therapist as a first step towards these identifications.

Sibling jealousy is a less difficult emotion for the student to comprehend. The arrival of a new baby represents a severe challenge to the child who is replaced in the most tender elements of his mother's care, by the newcomer. Very insecure children sometimes make violent and even murderous attacks on a baby brother or sister because they are unable to resolve their emotions. We have to grasp that these emotions are, or soon become, *complex* in the technical sense of this term, meaning that they are unconscious and still unresolved – foreign bodies in the psyche which have neither been extruded by conscious awareness and acceptance, nor assimilated, which situation would mean that they were dissolved in the psyche and thus no longer hurtful. Regressions, such as a return to wetting or soiling, a demand to return to the bottle, fretfulness or clinging to mother are not infrequent responses on the part of the anxious child. The child may go to the other extreme and become most loving towards the new baby and solicitous for his welfare. Herein we have the forerunner of the mothering or fathering instinct, but it may also be because he grasps that it is in this way that he can please his mother and thus retain for himself her love. The grasp here is an unconscious one and, therefore, both more real and more strong than if it were any intellectual appreciation of the circumstances. It may be that his aggressive feelings towards the baby have aroused sensations of guilt and fear. These are repressed and the child becomes overanxious about the baby. This is a frequent type of response. Again and again in the practice of psychotherapy with adult patients, no less than with children, one finds that the little one has felt rejected when the new baby has arrived, anxiety and hatred have resulted, aggressive feelings have been repressed and complex emotions of insecurity or unworthiness have motivated the anxiety states of adult life. One little girl, a week or two after the birth of a baby brother, dreamt that her mother was going to throw her into a cauldron of boiling water. She awoke in terror, rushed crying into her parents' bedroom, to be rebuked by her father for disturbing her mother – how blind is the adult world to the feelings of childhood! Whatever the reality of not unloving parents, unconsciously she believed this terrible state of affairs, so crushed must she have felt by the rejection which the coming of a new baby implied in her mind.

A strong, healthy child, whose mother is able to treat his difficulties with discrimination, is able to resolve the emotions of jealousy and in doing so his character becomes fortified. We need to find ways of giving to the child who is displaced by the new baby opportunities of feeling that he shares with his parents the possession of this child. He can be present at all sorts of nursing procedures; if he is old enough he can help, and occasions can be found for him to love the new baby, to caress him or do things for him. We feel that this sharing from the beginning will be the complement, in the case of the older child, to the policy whereby the new baby is given all the love and care of his parents just as if he were their only child, while this sharing attitude ensures for the older child the feeling of being loved and valued, as he has always been.

The latency phase extends from the age of six or seven to about eleven or twelve. In the successful solution of the Oedipus problem the child comes to accept the prohibitions of the loved parent and to dissolve his hatred for the rival parent of his own sex, thus making an adjustment in his relationship with both. The libidinal wishes are repressed, so that he emerges into the relatively sexless phase which is termed *latency*, and the energies which previously sought gratification are redirected to find an outlet in such forms as play, physical activities, romping around, showing off, and similar forms of acceptable behaviour. A few children, tomboyish girls among them, seem not to give up their sexual desires and they will masturbate during this time.

Because there is less preoccupation with the emotions of love, latency gives children an opportunity to learn. The boy's attachment to his mother wanes, and he becomes the grubby boy at school, whose interests are with his mates. The girl is less attached to her father as her interests turn to outside activities like games or dancing.

A child at this age is widening his social contacts and is developing a herd instinct in group play and in all sorts of associations with friends at school, in the street or in the countryside. Nevertheless, a general attitude of distrust and reserve is also characteristic of the period, and in accordance with the strong tendency to repression there is a limitation of imaginative life.

A substantial proportion of the children we see in a child guidance clinic come to us during the latency period. In treating them we have to remember that the strong sensual and love emotions have partially been repressed into the unconscious and that powerful resistances prevent their expression. Short of being able to win the child's confidence and to penetrate his resistances by means of the techniques employed in child analysis, a process requiring much skill and time, one will have to recognize that these defences cannot be overcome at this stage and that the child's deeper emotional problems can be dealt with only indirectly. This indirect dealing will depend on how far it is possible for the therapist to discover what is the nature of the child's problem. Even so, direct interpretation will often be unacceptable to the child, and it may be only by his attitudes, by his comments of a tangential character and by his influence on parental attitudes that the therapist can get across to the child.

A special difficulty arises in treating those anxious and inhibited children whose inner problem is one of sexual guilt. The therapist, seeing this, may be tempted to originate discussion of sexual subjects and thus to bring these anxieties into the open. But it is just here that the guilt feelings are so intense and the defences, therefore, so strong that the child dare not express these emotions. In the result the mention of sexual topics may do no more than increase his worry. The therapist who talks openly about these tabooed matters may, by doing so, ally himself with the forces of evil and may thus become frightening to the child, who may now see in him someone of whom his parents – at least the fantasied, idealized parents – would disapprove. Discussion of the facts of life, the facts of sex more properly called, is concerned with anatomical and physiological matters and tends thus to by-pass the sensual fantasies, so that we are at risk of missing our objective. The mark of the better therapist may be his ability to refrain from open talk of sex. We shall have a chance to discuss this further in the context of particular patients.

To some extent we may be able to get round the difficulty by taking the parents into our confidence. We may explain to the child's mother, if she is sufficiently receptive, something of the manner in which hidden sensual feelings are motivating her child's anxieties, and she may, in return, be able to give the therapist further insight into how her child gives expression to these feelings. It may be appropriate for her to initiate discussion with the child or by a change in her own attitudes she may come to express to him that she has a more enlightened view of these things. The therapist's wisdom may reside in his being aware of what is going on and yet holding back from open exploration of the emotional wound.

The *fears* from which children suffer are most likely to be prominent in the phallic phase or early in latency, such as fear of the dark, fear of being alone, fear of wolves or of men hiding in cupboards. Often they take the form of nightmares or night terrors. Fear of the dark may mean fear of being left alone, and in infancy the baby whose mother has put the light out can no longer see her and may therefore fear that she is no longer there at all. Fear of animals can be much the same thing in that it represents pictorial thinking, pre-verbal thought, and being alone may conjure up pictures of what might happen if one were left alone. Fairy stories may tell him that animals might attack him. The important thing, however, about such stories is that they are frightening situations told to the child by someone who loves him. Mother is introducing the child to the facts of existence in easy stages.

Fears of this kind are often evidence of super-ego activity. The man who threatens with cruel savagery or the beast which lurks in ugly ambush are no other than the child's unconscious fantasy of his own parents, vengeful for his oedipal lusts and aggressions. These fantasies bear no relationship to the actual attitudes displayed by parents. Although we believe that parental qualities will modify anxieties, the tolerant and understanding parent conveys no immunity, and the occasional unsympathetic or cruel parent can only be said to make things worse, but not to be the cause of the child's problem. Sometimes sounds of parental intercourse, heard by the child though not understood, result in anxiety-provoking fantasies.

One evening in early winter I was asked to go over to the general hospital to see a little girl who had been admitted in a state of acute terror. She was ten years old, she was the youngest of three children and in fact she had asked her mother to take her to the hospital. She clung to me in panic and begged me to stay with her. She said she was terrified, but could not explain the nature of her fear, and it was an emotion-raising experience to be clutched so violently by this attractive, frightened child.

Ellen had an I.Q. of 130; her terror, as we later discovered, had been a fear of death, but she had turns of not knowing where she was and of being frightened in such situations as assembly at school. Despite her intelligence she had difficulty with her lessons and this worried her considerably.

Ellen's home was by ordinary standards a satisfactory one, and in treatment sessions there was good reason to believe that sexual desires of an oedipal nature and masturbation anxieties were at the root of the problem, but it was apparent that no interpretations of this nature could be entertained. Supportive play therapy, with counselling for her mother, thus became the treatment of election. Eight years later Ellen returned to see me on account of phobic anxieties, and she then revealed the depth of the rifts which had existed within her family and the severity of the emotional stresses which she had suffered as a child, but of which she had been unable to speak at the time. Shortly afterwards she married.

Adolescence is a time when sexual emotions surge upwards in strength. There is a felt need to impress the opposite sex. The individual becomes conscious of his appearance and of his figure and dress becomes important. The strength of desire is matched by shyness of expression. The authority of the parents and of the social group forbids the full realization of the sexual instincts and this prohibition is reinforced by the super-ego within. The social and instinctual taboos have made sex 'bad'.

The adolescent tends to live much in his own world of fantasies, of daydreams, of images, of identifications and of hero figures. Matters of his concern are of great urgency to him, while his emotions are volatile and powerful. He may therefore be little interested in the practical realities of day-to-day living and find it difficult to concentrate on work or studies. He may have a need to create havoc in order to punish, to get affection, or even to be punished. In treatment it is necessary to understand behind his disordered behaviour into the realities of his need.

A schoolgirl aged thirteen was referred to the clinic. Her class had been instructed to write an essay in the form of a letter to a friend, asking the friend to pay a visit. This child wrote the letter to a boy and in the letter she said to him that he could sleep with her at night. She was very preoccupied with boys and had quite a collection of film stars, which she afterwards showed to me, but she was very shy. Her remark about the boy sleeping with her was not an indication of sexual precociousness or of 'naughtiness' but was simply the indication of her need to express her awakening desire for sexual love, and to have the existence of this desire accepted.

The diaries which some adolescents keep serve a similar purpose in providing an outlet for emotions. The diary is a sort of silent confidant where feelings can be expressed or secrets told without humiliation.

Daydreams serve a useful purpose in adolescence and may do so at some other times of life as well. They provide temporarily an escape from such harsh realities as the individual's own sense of inadequacy or simply the hard round of daily living. Often they are a wish fulfilment which not only gives satisfaction but which enables the adolescent, by working out in his imagination what he would like to do, to lay down some small foundation of future achievement. Play in childhood, hobbies in adolescence and creative imagination during the years of growth are forerunners of successful work and emotionally gainful recreation in adult life. Daydreams play a relatively small but useful part in treatment if we are able to get our patients to express them. Adolescents sometimes are able to do this, although sexual fantasies and those which the young person feels to be humiliating are hard to come by, but sometimes we can help by putting into words what the therapist believes to be the patient's thoughts. If the relationship is a good one the patient may accept these and even add to them. It obviously is unhealthy for an adolescent or an adult to live to excess in a world of fantasy, but in moderation daydreams can be a constructive element in mental life.

Anxieties about growing up can be very strong. A girl who has been told nothing about menstruation may be taken unawares and may suffer from feelings of fright and guilt or may imagine, as one of my patients did, that this meant that she had an illness that would require operation for its cure. Uninstructed boys sometimes have anxieties about seminal emissions. Self-deprecation arises from guilt over sex. The ego may retreat in the face of these pressures to a pre-genital stage. Examples are overeating in girls who stuff themselves or boys who develop dirty, untidy habits.

Hollingworth[15] told of an adolescent girl who, for about a year, was torn by a struggle between the wish to be a deaconess and the wish to be a circus rider. She used to spend mornings reading the Bible and sewing. The afternoons she employed in riding an old horse bareback around the common. This conduct was puzzling to her family, who feared she might be 'crazy'.

There is an underlying conflict between the old dependency upon the parents and a new desire for independence. There is an urge to rebel against father or mother and against the guilt feelings (super-ego) which are ultimately derived from their authority. The adolescent wants to defy authority. Because this defiance is due to a fear of sex he may in effect deny all love for his parents. There are swings from one mood to another; he may be aggressive or secretive and will avoid all intimate contact with his parents, sensing that he must not get too close. This denial of love for his parents and defiance of authority force the adolescent away from the family and into the group, which becomes all-important to him. Hero worship and an allegiance to the leader of the group or to its ideal represent displacements of love from father and mother: they also imply these identifications which mean that the boy in fantasy is the leader and himself possesses the qualities of success, altruism and achievement for which the group stands. Daydreams of success and greatness fortify the ego. This process of emancipation is necessary because continuing dependence on parental support in the emotional field stifles the development of mature, adult relationships, and the stunting of character growth which results is productive of some of the most resistant types of neurotic structure.

A young man who came to see me recently provided a characteristic example of this. He complained of insomnia and gastro-intestinal symptoms. He had allowed his life to be dominated by the necessity of helping to care for a mentally defective brother who was still at home, and by the obligation to support his ageing parents by remaining at home with them indefinitely, as well as by his financial contribution to the family economy. He was living a life restricted sexually and socially and his symptoms were the price he paid for the frustration to his ego that was involved.

High ideals and preoccupation with altruistic concepts are mingled with phases of feeling of the adolescent's own weakness. Stories such as 'Cinderella' or 'The Ugly Duckling' and religious sagas in which the humble person is elevated to greatness delight the imagination. Asceticism, tests of endurance, self-deprecation or even self-hurt, whether physical or in fantasy, are opposites of ego-inflation and are motivated by feelings of guilt or of rejection, the outcome of castration anxieties, by now, or course, fully repressed below consciousness.

The adolescent may see in religion or in some philosophy the answer to the problems of society and may decide to devote his life to the cause. Sometimes idealism and romanticism are lived out at a practical level in some form of voluntary service and adolescents may show that their feet are firmly planted on the ground. On the whole, however, adolescence is a time of instability, the ego being rather disorganized, so that its several, often conflicting, parts have still to be integrated into a harmonious whole – this after all is the problem which faces these young people and its resolution the objective they dimly have in view.

Narcissistic tendencies arise. Narcissism, or self-love, is appropriate to the phallic (genital) or even earlier stages of development, but in adolescence the ego, feeling that it cannot find love outside itself, may turn back into itself for its libidinous satisfactions. Relationships are made on a fellow-feeling basis, the other persons being identified with oneself; and from these identifications arises the tendency to ape others.

The adolescent questions the meaning of his own identity in relation to others. Uncertainties about the meaning of things worry him, he goes in for philosophical reflection about the stars, wonders about the origin and destiny of humanity, goes for long walks by himself, and he may appear to be solitary or withdrawn because he feels that he cannot share these preoccupations with anyone. Because of his doubts about himself he is sensitive to criticism, he may have difficulty in making good relationships, and those he does make may be brittle. Just as his feelings of isolation and his need to be loved or accepted may have brought him to join a group or gang, so his doubts may drive him away from it, and he may, therefore, decide to leave the group just when he seems to be most in need of its support.

Homosexual urges are normal in early adolescence before the sex instinct has become fully differentiated. In a sense these young people are repeating the childhood stage of narcissism which is characterized by the child's interest in his own body at the genital stage of development. Circumstances, such as segregation in one-sex schools and parental discouragement of mixing with the other sex, also play a part. 'Crushes' can be troublesome; they concern members of the same sex and involve jealousy in relation to the object of the crush. The varied nature of sexual expression which occurs in infancy led Freud to describe it as 'polymorphous perverse', and in adolescence we see a re-emergence of this variety of expression of love.

Adolescence creates mental problems that are difficult to solve and it is not, therefore, surprising that a number of children either become depressed or break down into a schizoid state of withdrawal. This also may be seen as regression to narcissistic levels. In the case of adolescents who appear schizophrenic we are justified in taking a much less grave view of the condition than would be the case with an adult patient, and schizophrenia should not be diagnosed in a young person unless considerable thought disorder is present, and not always even then.

We may classify adolescents as: (*a*) *Uncomplicated or simple*, being those who come naturally into mature sexual development. Wounds to their pride arise if sex relationships do not work out well. Their sexual feelings tend to be relatively crude. (*b*) A *neurotic*, but large and typical group, who display many of the defence mechanisms we have been discussing, such as asceticism, solitariness or idealistic surges. (*c*) A *mixed* group of young people who may change from one of the above types to the other. Groups or gangs may be divided into: (1) the *conforming* group, which is fostered by adults, and (2) the *tough* or *rebellious* group.

It can readily be seen how a youth or girl will, according to the circumstances both internal and environmental in which he finds himself, gravitate to one or other type of group. It is perhaps along such lines that we ought to seek the explanation of the recent upsurge of 'Teddy Boy', 'Mod' and 'Rocker' gangs, Hippies and the increase in delinquent trends. In many homes there has been a shift of emphasis away from caring for the family towards the importance of material benefits, and from this insufficiently loving atmosphere young people, seeking purpose in life, have gravitated towards association with others for whom, like themselves, life has little meaning other than to express the pervading sense of rejection which abides within them.

In the treatment of a large number of women and girls I have been impressed by the extent to which the girl's development is dependent upon feelings of being loved, valued and appreciated by her father. Far too many fathers are but dimly aware of this and do not realize the extent to which it is true that for healthy emotional growth their daughters need the sunshine of their interest and approval. A father may not have enough confidence in his own goodness to believe that his attitudes and attentions can be of such immense importance to his daughter. It is sometimes a part of our task to see a girl's father and to try to get the meaning of this across to him. What is the position of a girl who has lost her father by death? This is likely to be less damaging than is neglect by a living father and it is more easily compensated by the affections of a stepfather or another adult male relative.

CHAPTER IV
Emotional Illness that is Constitutionally or Organically Determined

Brain Damage. We already have touched upon the influence of physical and constitutional factors in causing symptoms.[16] When we make a diagnosis of brain damage in the child guidance clinic we mean that we believe there is sufficient psychological evidence to justify such a diagnosis in the absence of neurological signs or symptoms. There may have been resuscitation difficulties at birth, inability to suck or some other suggestive occurrence. The kind of symptoms we find suggestive are hyperactivity, inability to concentrate or abnormal emotional response such as constant demandingness and an incorrigible tendency to create disturbance. There *may* be some intellectual loss and the responses to the psychologist's test may be otherwise unusual. This sort of pattern, in the absence of family disturbance, if excessive and persistent makes a diagnosis of minimal brain injury seem reasonable and there may be some support from the E.E.G. in the form of minor dysrhythmias.

In treatment counselling for the mother takes first place. Its aim is to be supportive, to deal with any guilt feelings which she may have and to assist her, along with her husband, to accept this as a disability which is inevitable. The help of the pediatrician will be valuable in diagnosis and as regards treatment of any coincident physical disability. In handling the child the same psychological considerations apply as in the case of other children, while some extra allowance has to be made for emotions which cannot be controlled. Symptoms which cannot be controlled otherwise may be amenable to drug therapy and it will sometimes be necessary to admit the child to hospital for investigation of behaviour and of the capacity of a neutral environment to help him or in order to give the mother a break. The emotional risks of separating a young child from his parents may have to be weighed against other considerations.

The following case of a boy brought to see us at the age of four years two months, although bedevilled by a low intelligence, illustrates many of the problems. Michael was hyperkinetic, disobedient and rocked incessantly. He was said to have walked and talked at eleven to twelve months, although late with sentences, but when he came to the clinic the psychologist considered that his I.Q. was probably in the 50s. He liked to play with mud and water, but was difficult to amuse and could not concentrate. He had wandered from home, neighbours had complained of his behaviour and other children would not play with him. He suffered from a squint. He was the elder of two boys, delivery was normal, but the second stage of labour was long and he had a large cephalhaematoma.[17]

His parents' marriage seemed to be a happy one. The mother had so often been told that they should care better for Michael that she was actually relieved when told that we must consider the existence of brain damage as almost a certainty. Our suggestion was long-term contact with the clinic and that in the meantime regular medication be discontinued, but that the mother should have available a sedative such as chloral or tinct. camph. co., which she might let him have on nights when he was excessively restless. Schooling, nursery or otherwise, would have to be considered subsequently according to the circumstances from time to time.

Handicapped children, whether the disability is a mental or a physical one, may suffer emotionally to such an extent that they are referred to the clinic, and whether our help can most usefully be given through direct therapy or in counselling for parents will depend on circumstances. It has been my experience that some children so referred are so inhibited that to make a relationship with them is far from easy, and I believe that in practice we shall often have to be content to concentrate on helping those who are looking after them. To begin with there is the parents' burden of pain. Their sense of disappointment cannot be measured and too often it is reinforced by a feeling of personal failure or even of guilt. This was particularly evident recently in a case where a little girl had been badly burned and her mother, who was not entirely free from responsibility for what happened, experienced a great sense of guilt. There is a risk that if this guilt is not adequately handled it may unconsciously be turned into aggression towards or rejection of the child, at least at times of stress.

Denison, in handling the surgical treatment of a large number of cases of hare lip, has been impressed by the need for skilled emotional support to the mothers of children born with such disablements. This psychiatric care is, perhaps, a task which in view of the shortage of child psychiatrists, adult-orientated psychiatrists might be prepared to assume.

Bassa[18] has noted that the child with cerebral palsy has great difficulty in the perception and integration of tactile, visual, oral, kinesthetic, proprioceptive[19] and other stimuli, and that he may, therefore, misinterpret and even resent ordinary maternal activities such as fondling. His mother will then need help to understand and to adjust.

Allen and Pearson[20] showed that the child seems to adopt the same attitude towards his disability as his parents do. If they worry, he is likely to be distressed; if they are ashamed, he will be sensitive, too.

A child may be mentally subnormal, yet may flourish in a home where he is encouraged and receives praise for his help given in simple household chores. A withered leg may negative prowess in the games field, but its young possessor may revel in and succeed at carpentry or photography. A deaf child may find joy in the satisfaction of looking after a pet of which he is in charge. When, however, all is said and done, it is clear that prolonged or permanent physical handicap must produce emotional upset and this may be so deep as to modify a child's personality fundamentally. Such a child must sometimes experience a sense of irreparable loss and it would hardly be natural if he did not sometimes cry bitterly. The child must sometimes wonder, and fear, what the future holds for him. Perhaps we can help a little by a readiness to give some sort of answer to this difficult question and a willingness to discuss the problem sympathetically but realistically.

Inevitably these children are dependent upon the help of others, but it is also essential that they should learn to be independent. A sense of independence will counter feelings of inferiority, and in the end any real success in life, whether in the social, the economic, the matrimonial or the spiritual field is going to depend far more on what they can do for themselves than on what others can do for them. Handicapped children need to be trusted in the situations of everyday life and in such things as pocket money, possessions and hobbies. If it is otherwise they will come to feel that their parents lack confidence in them. In matters of personal privacy there is a danger that the legitimate needs of the disabled child may be forgotten. Every child is entitled to a degree of privacy and there are reasons why this may be of special importance in the case of those who have a disability.

A physical illness occurring in childhood may cause widespread emotional and sometimes intellectual difficulties. We were asked to see a boy of fifteen and a half, who, nine months earlier had had an illness, lasting a fortnight, and now regarded by the neurologist as having been encephalitis. He was the younger of two children. His mother was mildly anxious, his father's time with the family was limited, but both mother and father were devoted to their children. The marriage appeared a happy one and the home atmosphere warm and friendly. The boy's I.Q. was 99, he had some impairment of memory, and when we saw him he was still unable to attend school following his illness. He had concomitant strabismus, he was noted as having feminine contours and hair distribution and a pneumoencephalogram showed slight enlargement of the ventricles.[21]

He used to be interested in reading and television, as well as games, and he had had numerous friends, but he had lost these interests and had become a solitary boy, almost certainly due to the encephalitis. At home he was a 'mother's boy' and was fond of helping in the house. He came to camp with us and during the week there he appeared happy and was able to look after himself. On his day of orderly duty the other boys of the duty squad complained that he did not work. His contribution to the work was ineffective. It was obvious that in any employment he would need constant supervision and encouragement, but in general terms, his relationships with others were good.

Three years afterwards we heard that he was working in a dairy with long hours and poor pay and that he was anxious to hold down this job. There had been some mental and physical improvement and the only physical symptom remaining was uncertainty of balance. He remained solitary, but had joined a youth club; but as he could not ride a cycle or motor cycle he was not very acceptable in the club.

Epilepsy is often the cause of psychiatric symptoms. The malign capacity of epilepsy to cause difficulties of personality is one of its most characteristic features, as well as being one of the most difficult to explain. To those who live close to these children the recognition of this quality is inescapable.

Many epileptic children are in the low intelligence range, but not a few are bright and some are brilliant, while the disease may manifest itself as *petit mal* (pyknolepsy), as *grand mal* with typical seizures or in one or other of the more irregular forms. The amount and kind of personality disturbance also will vary. The child may be unhappy, fretful and anxious. He may suffer from a rather serious lack of self-confidence and this may produce or reinforce such secondary qualities as jealousy, resentment, aggression or inability to mix with others. He may be unduly demanding at home, excessively sensitive to criticism or intolerant of attention given to others. Behaviour disorder or delinquency may arise as an outcome of these personality problems, especially if the home environment has not been for the child a happy one or parents have lacked understanding. It will be apparent that none of these qualities is the peculiar perquisite of the child who has epileptic tendencies, but few, if any, epileptic children escape a measure of personality difficulty. We usually are justified in taking a fairly optimistic view of the outcome, especially in cases of *petit mal*, as these fits generally cease altogether. With *grand mal* we can expect a fair recovery rate, while those forms which produce confused or altered states of consciousness are rather more apt to persist. The personality problems are often the most refractory to treatment of all the characteristics of the malady, but with adequate handling they, too, can be appreciably ameliorated.

Drug treatment for the epilepsy is an obvious necessity and this is usually best prescribed with the help of the pediatrician or the E.E.G. expert. This, particularly in mild cases, can be expected to result in great improvement and often in permanent cure, but personality difficulties may persist. Although epilepsy is an organic, rather than purely psychological illness, psychological treatment is often necessary. Occasionally play therapy will be the answer, to be conducted as in the case of any other type of psychological problem, because in practice the motivations of behaviour difficulties are emotional – what is constitutional is the strong predisposition to their formation. In many cases difficulties will have arisen in connection with school and the educational psychologist is often able to assist in straightening these out, while the choice of school, or even a change of school, may require consideration. More important still, in most cases, is counselling for the child's mother and this is on the same principle as counselling in the case of other young children who have emotional difficulties.

Deafness in children creates problems in the emotional, the social and the intellectual field as well as resulting in secondary disturbances, of speech for example, and it may be confused with intellectual defect. Early recognition, in the first nine months if possible, is important, and if doubt remains the child should be treated as deaf. Deafness may be partial and it may be intermittent. In-patient observation may be necessary. Real sympathy is called for and one should speak clearly and reasonably loudly to such a child, but not shout. A good home background and very great patience on the mother's part are demanded. Teaching in a school for the deaf, which will often be residential, will become essential as the child grows older and there is scope for co-operation between psychiatrist, otologist and educationalist. Hysterical deafness can result in the failure of already established speech. Psychotic children may show functional mutism and deafness and sometimes they will respond to sound after a second or two.

Psychosis of childhood occupies a special place both from the etiological point of view and from that of treatment. Also known as *infantile autism*, it has to be defined as a clinical entity, and the practice is to be deprecated whereby conditions of severe maladjustment are included under the term *psychosis* because they are difficult to fit into any other category. The condition is in some way akin to schizophrenia of adult life, but we do not yet know sufficient to say how far the two can be equated. An element of withdrawal from adjustment to reality is a cardinal feature of childhood psychosis.

As is now fairly well known, a group of child psychiatrists surveyed the field in order to form some conclusion as to what were the principal features of the malady. Their findings have been published[22] as the nine diagnostic points and are, in brief, the following:

1. Gross and sustained impairment of emotional relationships with people.
2. Apparent unawareness of his own personal identity to a degree inappropriate to his age.
3. Pathological preoccupation with particular objects or certain characteristics of them, without regard to their accepted functions.
4. Sustained resistance to change in the environment and a striving to maintain or restore sameness.
5. Abnormal perceptual experience (in the absence of discernible organic abnormality).
6. Acute, excessive and seemingly illogical anxiety as a frequent phenomenon.
7. Speech either lost, or never acquired, or showing failure to develop beyond a level appropriate to an earlier age.
8. Distortion of motility patterns.
9. A background of serious retardation in which islets of normal, near normal or exceptional intellectual function or skill may appear.

It is inadvisable to diagnose psychosis unless the case substantially conforms to this description, and especially in respect of the failure to grasp the meaning of a relationship with parents or other people or the concept of toys (things) as capable of manipulation; yet there are children whose cases seem to occupy an intermediate position between normality and psychosis. It is almost as though they hovered on the brink, but did not fall into the psychotic abyss. These, for want of a better description, I have termed *schizoid children*.[23] Many workers and most parents of affected children prefer the terms *autism* and *autistic*. It is best to limit the word *psychotic* to describe those most severely affected, while *autistic* refers both to them and to the partially disabled group whom I describe as schizoid. Thus all children who suffer from characteristics of this type may be called autistic children.

The case of Arnold illustrates this difficulty of diagnosis. He was

CONSTITUTIONAL ILLNESS

referred at the age of five years and five months, the elder of two children, because of backwardness, especially in school. His mother, though anxious to co-operate, did not seem more intelligent than a very low average, but so far as we could assess the home was a happy one. Arnold was almost four when his sister was born. The story his mother told us was that he could talk at ten months, could repeat lines of verse at that age, that he could count up to twenty at two years old, but that he could do neither of these things now. He also used to draw better than he now could. At the age of almost three and a half his quiet temperament had changed and he became 'very naughty', but did not appear to have any illness. Parts of the story were conflicting. His mother went on to say that his performance at school was poor, but that he could learn quickly and knew the latest songs, but she could not teach him road sense and he would not mix with other children. He used to throw things at school, but now just sits quiet and will not do anything and if given crayons just breaks them up, so she told us. He no longer wet or soiled himself. He was jealous of his little sister and if Mother picked her up, he would say: 'Mum, I love you.' He certainly was not without affection for his mother and she said that he got on well with his father and played with him.

In the clinic he took my hand and came willingly to my room, where he spontaneously went to the sand tray and played happily. He spoke freely but indistinctly and he responded better to physical than to verbal contact. He could even smile, but his response was passive rather than spontaneous. Muscular co-ordination was reasonably good. His sand and other play seemed about the three-and-a-half-year level and pretty normal for that age. The psychologist assessed his I.Q. as being about 55. My finding was that this, at its face value, was a fairly straightforward case of mental subnormality, but in view of the pretty definite history of deterioration – about two years ago, his mother said, which was almost a year before his sister's birth if the dates were correct – this diagnosis could not be unequivocally accepted. The good contacts he made told against psychotic development and his good co-ordination was not in support of mental subnormality, in which muscular co-ordination tends to be impaired, but neither this nor the absence of any history of illness at the age of two, supported brain damage as a cause. Yet I fell back upon an unsuspected attack of encephalitis as best meeting all the data.

In view of these circumstances we asked a consultant in mental subnormality to see Arnold, a physician of long experience in the speciality, and the following is his report: 'I do not think there is any question about him being backward, but the causation seems to be what is in dispute. After the interview and from the history the mother gives, I would hazard a guess that this boy is psychotic, rather than the result of encephalitis, although this, of course, cannot be ruled out. He seemed to me to be listening on occasions as though he had auditory hallucinations, and the mother says that she has observed this on many occasions. He is very distractable, impulsive, and is quite unable to sustain interest or concentration beyond a few minutes.'

No specific treatment was suggested and when we saw him four years later, at the age of nine, he was emotionally detached and had a vacant expression, he talked with some freedom yet part of what he said was muddled, he was odd and yet in contact. He made a quite limited relationship with his mother. By that time he was attending the day school for educationally subnormal children and now, almost six years after we first saw him, he still has his place there. He is said to present difficulties, but the staff have hopes for him.

As regards the etiology of childhood psychosis two views have held the field, although they are not mutually exclusive. The first, the psychological or environmental theory, holds that babies who happen to be accepting and conforming may appear to be happy and contented even when left alone for long periods. Such a 'good' child may be left in his pram down at the end of the garden for hours, and the theory is that, assuming the child does not have a strong relationship-making capacity, he may gradually withdraw from emotional contacts, eventually becoming autistic. If this concept must be criticized on account of its incompleteness, it is still a useful pointer when we come to consider treatment.

The second view is that childhood psychosis must have a genetic origin in the same manner as is generally accepted in the case of adult schizophrenia. When one considers the number of children, afflicted by this malady, who come from excellent homes where they are loved and wanted, it is difficult to avoid the conclusion that here is a constitutional disorder which cannot, for the most part, be ascribed to environmental influence. It is not, however, supposed that the responsible cause is a dominant gene which would inevitably carry the malign factor, but rather that it is of a multifactorial kind, as appears to be the case with several other mental illnesses. This being so, it follows that environmental features will have an effect, and it may be in some cases a decisive one, in settling the matter as to whether or not a psychosis will actually develop or in influencing the degree of its severity. It has been suggested that a mother who is emotionally cool may have a child who becomes autistic. If this were so it would seem to favour the environmental theory, as the mother's coolness would be likely to arise from circumstances of her own childhood, but I know of no relevant study aimed to prove that such mothers are likely to have autistic children.

Creak[24] has been able to follow one hundred cases of psychotic children who eventually died and in several of whose brains demonstrable pathology was discovered at post-mortem. The full implications of this valuable work will be apparent only when wider studies are possible.

When we come to the treatment of infantile psychosis, or autism, we have at present no means of influencing whatever organic factors exist, so that we are dependent upon environmental therapy or psychotherapy. The latter, to have any hope of success, must be reasonably intensive, and it is unlikely that many child guidance clinics will be able to devote four or five interviews each week to the individual child, nor will every clinic have a therapist whose giftedness in understanding, patience and resilience is matched by the necessary training in analytical technique. Even so, these idealistic considerations should not discourage the therapist who is motivated to give what he can within the limitations of time available at an ordinary clinic, for worthwhile results have been achieved in some cases in this way. A cardinal consideration of treatment is that it should be early, and before much can be done in this direction it may be necessary to educate doctors, health visitors, parents and others to the need for referral to the child guidance clinic of every baby who displays a pattern of behaviour suggestive of autism and of every baby who, having progressed fairly normally up to a certain stage of development, ceases to do so or even regresses. A treatment attempt should precede a firm or final diagnosis because of the impossibility of assessing prognosis without some experience of treating the child. In treatment the first objective will be to enable the child to make some sort of contact with play objects and with the therapist. To do this may require inexhaustible patience in playing with a child who shows no understanding and makes no response or who perpetually goes off at a tangent. O'Gorman pointed out that it must be a monumental task to persuade a child to alter his pattern of thinking when he is unaware of any motivation, and perhaps has not even the mental tools necessary for doing so. Talking to the unrequiting child, handling him and sometimes lifting him playfully and affectionately, require both spontaneity and outgoingness as well as the capacity to imagine the child's emotional situation and to respond to its variations, and a real ability to care for handicapped children.

It is presumed, though direct evidence may be lacking, that the psychotic child passes through the same phases of emotional development as psychoanalysis has shown to be the lot of the ordinary baby, and that he will suffer the same frustrations, fears and aggressions, though the weakness of his inherent ego capacity may limit their impact. On this basis it will be the next objective in treatment to help the child to overcome these through the formation of an actual attachment to the therapist. To achieve this must require an extension of the process we have described – a capacity on the therapist's part to grasp the implications of these concepts for the uncommunicating baby and to give of herself to him in an outflowing of response, response which is channelled according to analytical concepts, while at the same time the therapist observes the rule of therapy that she does not become emotionally dependent upon the baby.

What part the child's mother will play in therapy must depend primarily on her own giftedness. The child who has become able to relate to the therapist will be able to relate to his mother and father, and will in time transfer his attachment if a worthwhile measure of recovery has been achieved. In many cases the absence of skilled therapeutic, as distinct from diagnostic, assistance will mean that the mother is quite the best available person to help her own child, and in such a case she may legitimately hope to receive from the child guidance clinic adequate counselling over an extended period.

If treatment is available the relative merits of its being on an outpatient or an in-patient basis may have to be considered. It is hard to justify, as a matter of election, the removal of an autistic child from an averagely good home. There may, however, be factors, such as sheer distance, or illness on the part of the mother, which render separation unavoidable, and it should then be a prime consideration to arrange for as frequent parental visits as are possible. The value of a 'break' for the mother who is overburdened is not to be forgotten. We may also consider getting someone, usually a relative, who can act as mother to both the psychotic child and in a sense to the child's mother also, to move into the home.

Hopes have been expressed recently that *behaviour therapy* in the form of *operant conditioning* will provide an advance on existing methods of treatment. The technique is, briefly, that the therapist first performs some action himself and at the same time names his action in words. When he has done this once or twice he gets the child to do it with him, rewarding the child with praise or with a suck of a lollipop or a small sweet. Once he has done this several times he persuades the child to do it alone, again rewarding the achievement each time. Eventually the child will perform the task on request, without the reward, and may even be taught to say words by this method.[25]

One is initially reluctant to support the use of a form of treatment

CONSTITUTIONAL ILLNESS

for a child which seems to be hardly different from the reflex training of an animal. Yet there may be more in it than this. The child may gain the glimmerings of a sense of achievement, a relationship between child and therapist may be fostered and speech achieved even in this reflex manner once begun may be improved. In any case, where a child is suffering from an illness which is as utterly destructive of personality growth as infantile psychosis is, it would seem a pity to rule out any method that gave even slight promise, unless it were positively harmful.

Hallucinations, even if they do occur, are not a prominent feature of childhood psychosis, although where adolescents are concerned the picture approximates much more closely to that typical of adults. We do, however, see the occasional boy or girl who complains of such phenomena, usually auditory, but without any other symptoms to suggest schizophrenia. In such cases, and especially if the child is living in a stress-provoking environment, we shall be justified in taking a guardedly optimistic view of the prospects. Attention should be paid to treatment in relation to the stress factors and the likely improvement to be derived from chloropromazine or a similar tranquillizer should be taken into account as part of the therapeutic programme.

Schizoid children[26] form a small group who display symptoms which, though not amounting to psychosis or autism, have an irrational quality about them and involve persistent impairment of adjustment to other persons and of attitudes to toys and other objects. Unnatural anxiety, inability to play with others or to respond to any scheme of activity whether in school or in the nursery and a quality of individualistic but unusual behaviour characterize them. One little boy found no interest in any of the toys, sand tray or paints in the clinic, but in one interview after another he devoted all his attention and his conversation to the plumbing under the playroom sink. He was too anxious, too restless and too disturbing in his non-co-operation to continue at school but after more than a year with an experienced occupational-play therapist he was able to attend a small school where special consideration could be given to his difficulties. What usually distinguishes these children from the truly psychotic is that they have at least a fair capacity to make love relationships with their parents and that, odd though their attitudes may be, they can converse with some degree of realism.

It has been the writer's policy, when such children are referred to the clinic, to make every effort to fit them into the category of emotionally deprived or anxiety-prone children and to conjure up from the history or the environment factors which may have motivated the origin of this anxiety. Alternative diagnoses such as mental subnormality or brain damage are rigorously eliminated by intelligence testing, pediatric examination, and where indicated, such special tests as E.E.G. But when all this has been done there remain a small number who qualify for inclusion in this oddly reacting, schizoid group. Their treatment is along the same lines as that which has been outlined in the case of autistic children.

Uncommon or not easily recognized types of *physical illness* or of *congenital abnormality* can present a pitfall in the child guidance clinic where the psychiatrist may not have had pediatric training, the other members of the staff are non-medical and screening by family doctor or school medical officer has been inadequate. Cases we have had recently to consider have included one of craneostenasis and oxycephaly, two involving the disorders of sexual development involved in Turner's syndrome and Kleinfelter's syndrome, hypsarrhythmia or salaam spasms with abnormalities of E.E.G. as the keystone of diagnosis, and one or two of the metabolic disorders of childhood which, to those who are uninitiated pediatricwise, may simulate neurosis. The clear inference is that every child psychiatrist should, as part of his training, have spent some time in a pediatric department. Failing this one needs to have the eye that is ever open to pediatric possibilities. Anything that is odd in the child's appearance, symptoms which somehow do not conform to what can be fitted into psychiatric symptomatology, locomoter difficulties, undue fatigue – these may have significance in the field of organic medicine. It is a cardinal value in child guidance that we aim to insure against missing the possible physical origin of any symptom, and this responsibility must inevitably rest on the shoulders of the psychiatrist, who is the only medical member of the clinic's team of workers.

Hyperkinetic Children. Hyperkinesis or overactivity is sometimes spoken of as though it were a syndrome on its own, as indeed it may occasionally appear to be. It is of more practical value to regard this kind of behaviour as a symptom of disturbed emotional functioning. Some cases are due to minimal brain damage, although either can exist without the other. Sometimes hyperkinesis is the form taken by psychotic development; the constant movements and overactivity seem meaningless, and the child's relationships with those around him and his play with toys and other materials purposeless. Adequately staffed day-hospital units are likely to play a large part in the treatment of such children in the future, with residential accommodation where necessary, and in the case of older children special residential schools or special day schools. Where such facilities are not available treatment sessions in the clinic plus counselling interviews for mother or for both parents, or in some cases counselling alone, may provide the bare essentials of therapy. Such a service is not to be taken lightly; it requires time no less than skill and should be backed by the consultative facilities of a pediatric hospital. If the staffing of these units can include a fully trained child psychotherapist, so much the better. Members of staff should be flexible personalities, chosen for their freedom from complex motivation. They should have opportunities for training in the understanding of children; and the contribution of the children's psychiatrist, in addition to whatever direct therapy he provides, will be to get across to them the significance of a disturbed child's actions and to assist them in the handling both of the children's behaviour and of their own, related, emotional problems.

In those cases where the available evidence is not such as to justify us in entertaining the suspicion that there is brain damage or that the child is psychotic, the explanation of the child's overactive or excessively naughty behaviour must be sought in some area of disturbed child-parent relationship. If the nature of this can be elucidated, if the mother can be enabled to grasp what is happening in her child's emotional life, and if she can give more of her time and interest to him, we are likely to be well on the way to an eventual solution of the difficulty. In all these cases – the organic, the psychotic and the emotional – it is important that we should visualize the deep reality of the parents' plight, their need to be helped to understand and to be supported, and to be freed through the relationship quality of the counselling sessions from some part of the load of complex-motivated anxiety and guilt which they themselves are harbouring.

CHAPTER V

Disturbances Characterized by Free-floating Anxiety

There is a unity in treatment in child guidance which takes but limited cognizance of the symptom from which the child is suffering. Thus it comes about that two children, one of whom has been stealing, while the other wets his bed, may both be treated in much the same way; whereas two other children, both of them referred for, shall we say, school phobia, may be treated by different methods. Diagnostic labels, therefore, are by no means closely related to forms of treatment. Yet there are a number of broad tendencies which enable us to connect certain types of symptom with probable causes; and if we are thus helped to understand the cause we shall also be assisted in planning treatment. It is therefore worth while to take a look at the syndromes more commonly met with in the psychiatry of childhood. A question which we often have to ask ourselves in the psychotherapy of adult patients is: 'What is the emotional meaning of this symptom for this patient? Why does he have this particular symptom?' To no lesser degree these questions are relevant in the treatment of children also, and the question may be rephrased as: 'What is this child achieving by behaving in this particular way?'

Anxiety States
When we have attempted, in the clinics in which I work, to classify our children according to symptoms, anxiety states have always been the largest single category, though some workers claim pride of place for behaviour disorders. This is in part because the term is a wide one and because anxiety is so universal anyway. Anxiety states include the cases of those children who are unhappy, those who are insecure and timid, those who are rejected or deprived, those who are poor social mixers, some children who are very jealous and some who are aggressive. We may take along with them a number of symptoms which would, in the case of an adult, generally be regarded as hysterical or conversion symptoms. Thus we have emotionally motivated pain, usually abdominal, vomiting, anorexia, paresis, sensory manifesta-

tions other than pain, while recurrent minor illness in childhood must come under suspicion for possible psychological origins.

Hysteria is believed to take its origin during the fourth and fifth years of life, when genital anxieties are prominent and defence is by repression. If we regard it as a malady in which psychosomatic symptoms bind the anxiety, so that the latter is no longer free-floating, and in which a personality disorder arises involving a high degree of self-centredness and a marked tendency towards projections of feelings on others, so that the patient's hostile emotions are attributed to them, then we are justified in claiming that childhood behaviour disorder is not hysteria and that psychosomatic pains in childhood are not hysterical. Occasionally we see an older child who appears to be developing the characteristics of the adult malady.

An eight-year-old boy was referred because of periodic 'inability to see'. From the age of three he had been frequently under medical supervision for 'ears', 'eyes', undescended testicles and other ailments. He was the eldest of three children, both parents were affectionate, but father was sharp-tempered and he was afraid of him. No specific treatment was necessary. Over a period of nine months he was seen six times at the clinic and recovery appeared complete.

A girl of thirteen, of average intelligence, complained of persistent pain in the ears. She was unhappy and had few friends because of her supercilious attitude towards others. She was the elder of two children and her mother said the family was a happy one, but the family doctor had adequate reason to believe that the father was a bully. The girl complained bitterly of the pain, the E.N.T. department had examined her carefully with negative results, but she had little insight. After she had been attending our clinic for more than two months her mother sent us a curt letter to say that her daughter did not wish to come any more. Some years later our social worker paid a visit and her enquiries left little doubt that the girl had made a good recovery from the pain and that there had been an improvement in her general bearing and in her relationships. It is impossible to say just what, if anything, our intervention did for her. She may have gained some insight into the fact that this was *her* problem and not entirely the result of forces outside her control, and parental and other family attitudes may have been favourably influenced by the change of approach from the organic to one with a psychological slant.

A simple fear of leaving mother is a common manifestation of anxiety. Negatively toned symptoms, such as disobedience and destructiveness, are the obverse side of the same coin. In planning to treat these cases we may justifiably expect to find that attitudes on the mother's part are, if not actually causing the symptoms, subtly fostering them, and in treatment as much attention should be paid to parental rôles as to the child's own motivation.

Eileen was referred to us by the pediatrician when she was nine and a half years of age. Her I.Q. was 146. The complaint was that for more than two months she had suffered from abdominal pain and from fears, and that she had refused to be separated from her mother. She was tense, slept poorly and had always been nervous of some phenomena such as thunder. She was described as miserable at school. At our suggestion that she should leave her mother in the clinic waiting-room she howled with fear and rage and most of the psychiatrist's interview (at which he had to allow her mother to be present) was a howling match interspersed by angry expressions – 'I'll stay with you' – and demands to know why she should have come – 'What's the use?'. She agreed, however, to play skittles and she even smiled.

Shortly afterwards the doctor was able to see Eileen's father. He was twenty-five years older than his wife, he gave the impression of good family relationships, said Eileen would sit on his knee if she was alone with him, but that she was wont to upset her mother and would then worry because she had done so. But her mother had said: 'Eileen is like her father and they loathe one another.'

Eileen was the elder of two girls and her sister was described as being bright and attractive and as father's favourite. Eileen had been a tiny baby and in the first few weeks she got insufficient nourishment, as her mother's milk was scant. There had been no other obviously traumatic episodes in her early life, but at the age of five she was suddenly whipped off to have appendicectomy and two years later she had tonsillectomy. Her father said that she steeled herself against this, but that it 'took a lot out of her'. In babyhood there were no toilet training or weaning difficulties, but at the age of six she had been upset by there being a pail type of lavatory at school. She said to her mother once: 'I wish I could be like Janet and Louise: they go out to play. And I wish I could let you go and enjoy yourself.' Neither from these circumstances nor from the therapist's findings were we able to formulate a clear idea of the etiology of this anxiety. No indication of any hidden family problem ever emerged. Sexual ideas did, however, and it seems likely that fear and confusion concerning the emergence of new personality forces within herself were her nuclear difficulty. A series of nine therapeutic interviews was followed by a satisfactory result.

The first interview, which the therapist had reason to fear might be a difficult one, was conducted easily by Eileen herself. She went to the lavatory, played with animals, with a castle and with dolls' furniture, said she was a tomboy and liked to play with boys, adding that she had made friends with one boy 'with difficulty because they're so shy'. Afterwards she remarked on the change in herself, to the effect that she felt easier, and she added that she disliked changes, preferring things that were old and traditional. No specific interpretations were made, but Eileen had exteriorized material in a way that was itself beneficial.

In the next interview she played with the dolls' house. 'Sometimes I'm a baby when I play with the dolls' house.' She said she liked to have a water pistol to squirt at workmen and that twice they had taken it from her. Soon she went to the lavatory and told the therapist that she had diarrhoea from eating grapefruit. Asked about the words used for lavatory functions she said they were 'wee' and 'big'. At school, she said, the lavatory wall was being taken away and the girls had to be careful that boys did not see them. This was accepted, the therapist considering it safer to take what was given rather than to risk disturbing the relationship by pressing. Something might have been said about the girls' desire to see the boys in their lavatory and about the obvious symbolic significance of the water pistol, the interesting fact that she had gone to wee-wee (diarrhoea?) just after talking about squirting (wee-weeing) with the water pistol. She had said herself that she was a tomboy and one could have referred to the feelings of jealousy and desire that spring from the male's possession of a penis. One has just to decide how much to say and what to omit. After this there was some 'pretend' play, and finally sand play when Eileen said that Daddy was such a baby at the seaside because he played with sand castles. It is the strength rather than the ambivalence of her relationship to her father that is important, and it is significant that calling her father a baby reveals her awareness of the fact that she herself is growing up.

In a later interview Eileen buried a pig and a man and said they had been buried for ages and might be discovered by an archaeologist, and the therapist referred to the circumstance that people long ago had emotions similar to those we have now. In one interview she chose to play draughts with the therapist. One of the draughtsmen was missing and a two-shilling piece was used instead. The therapist gave this to Eileen afterwards, but she asked her mother to tell him at the next interview that she was afraid lest he do this again if they played once more. Unconscious sexual fantasies underlie this fear. The therapist said that draughts was one way of coming close to him. One part of her wants both to possess the therapist and to belong to him and yet she was afraid to take money, which is like taking a bit of the therapist, just because that means that they do belong to each other. These interpretations she was able at least partially to grasp. A second game raised relationship material regarding her desire to win, her unwillingness to accept any concession from the therapist and her attitude to his winning. Subsequently she painted and in her criticism of what she had done she displayed her strong need to be critical, even denigrating, of her own achievement. More illustrative still was a picture she drew at home for the therapist and which she sent to him through the post, of a pony, standing alone in open country, its mane blown wildly in the wind. This was so much a picture of her fantasy of herself, standing back to the wind, braced against the vicissitudes of life which she could just manage to prevent from overwhelming her.

The remaining interviews were less productive and a desire to stop treatment emerged. The picture she had sent through the post was discussed. Eileen recited to the therapist a poem in the bathroom at home, which enjoined the occupant to keep the bathroom clean, not to waste the soap and so on, and this was probably in line with much of the super-ego pressure that existed in this conventional British household. When her short series of interviews ended Eileen was still inhibited as regards freedom of expression and she was still a little too polite and too apologetic. The therapist felt, however, that she had been helped considerably and that perhaps the meaning of the change was that she could now feel more independent and would feel confident enough to do some things on her own.

Before Eileen first came to the clinic it had been arranged within the family that she should go to a boarding school after the following summer. In the clinic we accepted this plan and it was adhered to. After she had been at the boarding school for one term we saw her in the holidays, when both she and her mother were happy about how things had turned out. More than eight years after her initial interview an enquiry elicited the information that she was shortly going to a college of art in the metropolis, that she was happy, that she had several friends and that she was free from problems except such as arose from her artistic temperament.

Nightmares, night terrors and *sleepwalking* are common symptoms, which for treatment purposes we may consider together. Nightmares are bad dreams which the child tells afterwards to his mother, and if these are an isolated symptom, sympathetic encouragement is likely to be sufficient. If for one reason or another treatment is indicated, it will follow standard lines. The dreams may then be of help towards understanding the child's unconscious anxieties, but direct interpretation may be inappropriate. To some extent bad dreams are a normal part of life and it usually will be wise to avoid making a mountain out

ANXIETY STATES

of a molehill by suggesting that actual therapy is desirable. It seldom is.

Night terrors are episodes in which the child shouts, cries and looks terrified but does not waken up, and of which he remembers nothing in the morning. It is virtually impossible to waken the child. Ordinarily the best treatment is to discuss the situation reassuringly with the parent and at some length. By thus enabling parents to handle the problem dispassionately and with confidence we can deal satisfactorily with the symptom and the parents know that the clinic is available should they wish to return.

Sleepwalking is dealt with in the same way. Parents are naturally concerned lest the child who walks in his sleep may injure himself. I have once known of a child getting so far as to be hanging by his arms outside an upstairs window while still asleep. Real accidents must be exceedingly rare, but such precautions as fastening windows are reasonable.

The opportunity of witnessing a night terror does not frequently come the psychiatrist's way, but the writer had this experience a few years ago when we took to camp with us a boy who was then subject to these disturbances. On the night in question and shortly after going to sleep he began to call out in obvious distress and to be restless in his bed. What was so striking was that he was quite unrousable and it was easy to appreciate how parents, faced with such a situation, could become alarmed. We removed the boy to another tent by carrying him across the field and put him back to bed, but he continued to speak out in apparent terror and it was still impossible to rouse him or to establish any contact with him. Reassurance was thus of no avail and the whole episode lasted for about half an hour, after which he became quiet and continued to sleep peacefully.

Overeating is an interesting symptom because of the fundamental relationship between suckling and loving. We are likely to find that the child who eats greedily or excessively is, in fantasy, going to the breast, devouring, so to speak, as much love as he can possibly get. Such children are likely to be, in some way, starved of love, or at least to have an unconscious fantasy of being insufficiently loved. This is a good example of the meaning of a symptom and is a guide towards treatment.

Obesity. Young children cannot be expected to co-operate in dietary restriction, so that a mother's ingenuity in devising a low carbohydrate diet for the whole family is the best hope.[27] Older children, aware of their problem, can co-operate if given support. The value of dexamphetamine is established but justification of its use is questionable. A psychological orientation towards the child and towards relationships within the family, on the part of the medical adviser, will not be misplaced.

Thumb-sucking and *nail-biting* are to be regarded as more or less normal forms of sensual satisfaction. Sucking of the tongue is a more difficult problem, said to be commoner in mental defectives.[28] In the case of the two former, unless they are severe, it seems a pity to worry about them or to bother the child. In troublesome cases we should consider the possibility of emotional stress or want of satisfaction. One intelligent boy sucked his thumb till the age of twelve despite discouragement from the family. One day, during a casual family chat, someone offered him sixpence to stop the habit. From that day to this – and twelve years have elapsed – there has been no repetition of the habit. Dental surgeons have made us aware of the risk of lower jaw deformity in persistent cases.

Rocking or *rolling* and *jumpy* or *jerky movements* are another form of self-gratification and are, therefore, antidotes against anxiety. *Head banging* is a more severe form, said to occur mostly, though not exclusively, in subnormal children. Our policy in handling these problems is firstly to exclude organic factors and subnormality as possible causes, and if we have a green light in these respects to assess the child's circumstances within the family. The time of origin of the symptom may be important in relation to some other occurrence, such as having to leave the cot in order to make way for a younger sibling. There may be evidence of frustration earlier in relation to feeding or the child may display some other evidence that he does not receive an adequate amount of love and attention. Often we shall draw a blank in all these enquiries. In that event our most useful contribution will be in counselling the parents as regards their own anxieties and their unconscious guilt in relation to the child. In this way, being freed to devote themselves to their child, unencumbered by worries, they are likely to give him something of themselves that was lacking previously. Even if the symptom persists for some time it will no longer undermine the mother's equilibrium and we can be confident that improvement will set in in time.

Hair-pulling is a relatively uncommon complaint and unless it is a symptom of organic disorder is likely to indicate a disturbing degree of emotional stress. Occasionally a large proportion of the child's hair has been pulled out. The significant question is: Why is this child unhappy? Play therapy may be of value in handling the case, but we must look closely at the home circumstances and at the relationships which have developed there. One little girl, aged five and a half when she first came to us, whose mother's attitudes towards her were marked by much ambivalence, did not respond well to play therapy.

We therefore decided that the environment of a residential school for nervous children would be beneficial, and this turned out to be the case.

Breath-holding attacks, though uncommon, are not exactly rare and are one of the most alarming manifestations of interpersonal tension in childhood.[29] Fear, frustration, anger or even some physical upset may set off an attack. The child's breathing stops for what seems a dangerously long period and, exceptionally, unconsciousness or a convulsion may supervene. The diagnosis will usually be easy, but confusion with epilepsy or laryngismus stridulus, an organic symptom of latent tetany, can occur. It seems a pity to do unnecessary investigations unless there are real grounds for doubt. Treatment will follow the standard line of enquiry into family stress. It is parental anxieties and emotional attitudes, even more than those of the child, which will require our attention; and in practice it will usually be treatment interviews with the mother, and not forgetting father's influence, that are most important. Catzel[30] from his experience in the Transvaal, considers that iron deficiency is the cause of breath-holding, and also of sand-eating.

Croup is a form of laryngeal spasm, regarded by Soddy[31] as a night-time panic state, but it can also occur by day as a spasmodic cough. Maternal reassurance to the child, backed by an attitude of understanding confidence in the mother's own mind, is likely to be the best therapy. The condition may recur over a long period. A warm fruit drink will be comforting to the child.

Fainting attacks can occur in girls or boys of any age, but in my experience their significance is greatest in teenage girls, in whom they usually are symptomatic of anxiety about growing up. Treatment meets strong resistances, corresponding with the degree to which this highly charged sexual material is repressed.

It is my practice to explore lightly with these girls the anxieties which they are repressing in the hope that the girl will accept the existence of her problem and so be able to come to terms with it. If the resistances are too strong and therapy, as a result, too upsetting to be admissible, I then prefer to leave the young person in the hope that time will bring maturity and that the explanations which the brief therapy has provided will open the door slightly to eventual insight. I believe it is a mistake to give drugs to these patients, unless quite temporarily in order to tide them over some ordeal such as an examination. Nearly always one finds that the mother's anxieties are reinforcing the child's symptom and there often is a sort of unconscious collusion between the two with a view of keeping the girl in a state of infancy. It is therefore of vital importance that the mother's problem should receive attention and the social worker's efforts may, in favourable cases, achieve wonders in ameliorating the relationship between mother and child. In selected cases the psychiatrist may prefer himself to see the mother instead of treating the girl.

Daytime fears, fear of illness, of animals and the like is a relatively infrequent reason for referral to child guidance. It is not usually necessary to take a serious view of this sort of thing and the sheet anchor of treatment is an understanding but confident attitude on the part of parents. By good fortune, perhaps, it has been my experience that children who suffer from these fears usually come from satisfactory homes. One can generally be reassuring to parents that these states of fear usually clear up comparatively quickly. At the same time it is a good part of the plan if we can take the boy or girl for a fairly short term of therapy, which is mainly of a relationship and reassurance kind and may, of course, include play.[32] Where the fear is of a single object, such as some animal, and is persistent, behaviour therapy may be the best answer, and one can ask a colleague who is familiar with this kind of treatment to undertake it, unless one wishes to learn the techniques oneself.

Obsessional illness presents a far more difficult problem. Like most other neurotic problems, this is a manifestation of anxiety, and in the case of younger children, at least, the obsession is not yet completely separated off from the anxiety, so that there usually is a strong anxiety or fear component present. Where older children are affected the illness approximates to the adult pattern of obsessional acts or compulsive thoughts, and overt anxiety is less. The origin of obsessional illness is believed to be somewhere about the three- or four-year level, when pre-genital factors are dominant and defence is mainly reactive. The illness represents a reaction formation as defence against the forbidden libidinous desires.[33]

Griselda was fifteen and a half when she came to see us on account of compulsive washing of hands, clothes and hair, symptoms which had begun about three years previously. The family was a relatively colourless one, living in a respectable area of the city, father a civil servant, conscientious, concerned for his family and straightforward in his approach, and mother a friendly, accepting individual who herself suffered from obsessional symptoms, having to check and recheck that she had turned off the gas. There was an elder brother with whom Griselda was in a good deal of conflict and who teased her. She was socially shy and did not have a boy friend, though anxious to have one. Educationally she did well in the secondary modern school. We soon discovered that she did not get on well with her father, who found her behaviour trying and who, she felt, did not understand the 'younger generation'. The therapist visited Griselda's home in order to meet her father and to have a talk with him, and this he found helpful.

In the second interview the therapist decided to ask what she would like to do when grown up, having it in his mind that sex and marriage might be included in the programme. Griselda said she would like clerical work and would like to go abroad, explaining that she felt conditions in this island to be cramped. She added that she got on well with people, although she had difficulty in meeting strangers, as she felt that they could talk whereas she could not. Attempting to explore her difficulties further, we found that she was fond of clothes and could not afford as much as she would like. This was discussed in relation to her father's income. She then got on to talking about her mother's irritability and fussiness and her father's harsh misunderstanding of her illness. At this point the therapist said that Griselda did not look happy and it came to light that she did not like coming to the clinic because, she said, she did not like the therapist's questions. It was, therefore, tied up between the girl, her mother and the therapist, that he would see her father – the visit to which reference has already been made – and that we should leave Griselda to carry on under her own steam, if that was what she really wished, while her mother and the social worker might have such contact with each other as seemed to them to be appropriate.

Some days afterwards her mother phoned to say that Griselda would like to return to the clinic. At the next interview the therapist asked about dreams and Griselda told the following dream which she had had recently. She was visiting her girl friend in a back-street house and was asked to stay for tea. The girl's brother came in and was horrible; he chased her and she ran for the bus. There was now a war and there were German officers and a white car with 'Surgeon' painted on its side, and she seemed to have done something wrong and was bundled into the car while people tried to rescue her. She was taken into a place like a cafeteria and was serving soldiers. She then awoke. Griselda interpreted the girl's brother as her own brother. Her feelings were discussed with the therapist and she accepted his remark that her brother was a 'dirty dog'. The therapist interpreted the girl's brother also as representing other boys, the bad and the dangerous in boys and her own fear of growing up. The German officers he interpreted as being her father, who fitted this part rather well. Griselda interpreted the surgeon as the therapist and the therapist said, 'I am afraid so!' He spoke about how the surgeon was very bad and very good and of her ambivalent feelings about him. The people trying to rescue her represent her desire to continue as she was and not to have to face up to her problems. The therapist also explained her serving soldiers in the cafeteria as her fantasy of looking after her own husband and children later on in her own home.

In the next interview the therapist worked round to asking more about relationships at home. Everyone was trying to be nice to her now and she resented this from her father and wanted him to leave her alone. She agreed with the therapist that she was now in some way afraid of his loving her. She remembered how long ago he used to take her out on Sundays and his subsequent annoyance at the inconveniences her neurosis caused hurt her. She had always been fond of Mum, who was the one who got the blame if she was 'fed up'. A boy friend had asked her out, but she did not want to go, as she felt he was not genuine.

She painted a picture of a great rock overhanging the shore and a sea of green, white-crested waves. She accepted the interpretation that the stormy sea represented life's difficulties and the rock love and a husband. She had a dream in which she and her friends wanted to climb into a castle. Her mother said, No, so she just watched her friends go up. Later they fell. The therapist said that this seemed to mean wanting to do things that others did, but that something inside said they were bad or dangerous. This something was not really her mother, but was a feeling that had been built into her from attitudes she thought her mother and father had taken long ago. Relationships with boys could be a case in point and the fact that her friends fell in the dream could mean that punishment would follow such 'bad' behaviour. She seemed able to assimilate this interpretation. After a pause the therapist asked about feelings. Griselda asked what feelings and the therapist said, 'Any.' She then said that she had not been so 'fussy' lately, for what reason she did not know, was not washing her hair so often and was sleeping better. The therapist asked about present anxieties and she raised the issue of her forthcoming holidays and the prospects of a job when she left school. Three interviews subsequent to this were devoted largely to discussion of present boyfriend relationships and to consolidating what we had gained.

Sixteen months after this Griselda came by invitation. She had in the meantime left school and had a good job. She said that her neurosis did not improve during the time when she was coming to the clinic nor until nine months after she ceased to come, when she suddenly grasped that all this washing was silly, and that she had been well since then. This raises the difficulty which bedevils us in any survey we do of past patients because there is no certainty that any improvement achieved was due to the therapy undertaken. In the present case there are adequate grounds to believe that the treatment was necessary and at least a strong likelihood that it played a part in the outcome.

By no means all our obsessional cases are so easy to treat. The younger ones especially are apt to suffer from acute and persistent anxiety which is often heightened by therapeutic effort. Admission to a hospital ward for the treatment of child psychiatric patients is sometimes necessary to provide a stable emotional background, to relieve domestic tension and to provide sufficient play therapy sessions. In severe cases the use of tranquillizing drugs can be a valuable remedial measure.

An obsessional illness in a younger child will involve the mother in a very testing situation and she may require a great deal of help from the social worker. Even if the child's neurosis arises in some measure from parental anxieties – which may in part be corrected during the child's treatment – it stems in reality from deeply placed guilt feelings regarding sexual fantasies, and the defences against their emergence into consciousness are quite strong.

In psychotherapy interpretations are best restricted to what the child is reasonably well able to assimilate. In the case of Alistair, aged seven years and four months, we had evidence of such feelings – from an incident of sex play with a little girl, from his reaction of anxiety and aggravation of his obsessional symptom of hand-washing following an erotic scene on television and from a dream – but interpretation had to be very cautious. The strength of the parental reaction to the incident with the girl was also revealing. Indeed, we pay much attention to the anxieties and attitudes of the parents and particularly those of the mother, both to those problems which she has in her own right, so to speak, and also those which concern her feelings towards her child. As a preliminary to treatment it is useful to find out from the child's mother what are the family names for the sexual organs and for the excretory functions.

Inability to go to sleep at night may be due to the fact that when mother is no longer visible the baby fears that he has lost her. An arrangement such as leaving on a light, leaving a door open or calling upstairs may provide the necessary contact. Often it is in reality the mother's own attitude which brings about the difficulty. She may even waken the child by her fussiness to see that he is still breathing or by her own anxieties she may abet the child in his resistance against being left alone.

With children who are a little older one has to counsel parents towards a midway course of understanding that the child is anxious and may be afraid, but at the same time firmness in insisting that he should have regard to his parents' wishes. It will sometimes be necessary for the parents to allow the child temporarily to come into their bed, but he should know that this is a special concession and not a right. If parents will take the trouble to allay the child's fears when that is necessary and yet to exert control where they should, this kindly discipline will achieve results. Occasionally a few sessions in the clinic with the child, wherein an attempt is made to elucidate his fears with him, may be an advantage.

Depressed Children
In adult psychiatry the concept of an endogenous form of depression is widely accepted; besides which, many depressed states which are not truly endogenous or not genetically determined are none the less the result of unconscious factors, usually of a complex kind and relating to experiences of childhood, but sometimes to matters in the more immediate environment. The nuclear factor is sometimes the loss of a loved object, which may be something within the child himself or may be a part of him; or it may be a loved one in his immediate circle or something important in his environment. The recognition of this factor and the discovery of the nature of this loved object may require a very careful and insightful appraisal of the child's environment and of his emotional responses to it. In children up to the age of twelve or thirteen endogenous depression appears to be quite uncommon. We do, however, see the occasional girl or boy who is dull and unhappy, who complains or withdraws, who may even show delinquent behaviour and who can co-operate little at home and perhaps not at all in the clinic. If invited to come for treatment these children may express a desire not to do so, but a striking feature of their illness is that they may rapidly recover after months of being depressed. There is little we can do for them and in my experience drugs have not helped them much. Yet it is important to keep in touch and one feels that drugs should be employed.[34]

A much larger group of our child patients are those who are unhappy from environmental causes. Although unconscious factors are a major etiological influence, depressed children are children whose anxieties are so great as to have made them unhappy, and these anxieties are related to the environmental situation and are a reflection of the emotional relationships existing at home. Even the rare cases of suicide in children are best to be regarded in this light. Naturally one would breathe no hint of such an opinion to parents who had suffered the loss of a child in this way.

Therapy, correspondingly, must concern itself with relationships. Feelings of unworthiness, guilt, resentment or injured pride and the effects of an unresolved Oedipus situation are important issues, but in children these are more often capable of resolution through an adjustment of relationships within the family than is the case with older patients. I have been impressed by the strength of the aggressive component in some of these depressions and this sometimes accounts for delinquency.

In those cases where anti-depressive drugs are indicated amitriptyline, parstelin, tofranil and nardil are among those, one or other of which we may employ. The usual precautions as regards the non-use of alcohol, or in the case of parstelin and nardil the non-eating of cheese, as well as the possible risk if another drug is taken concurrently, have to be adopted. I have never used E.C.T. for anyone under sixteen and its employment should never be considered unless all else has failed. Yet it is the emotional handling of these depressions which is the sheet anchor in treatment and too ready resort to drugs is inappropriate.

Suicide clearly originates in anxiety and unhappiness, but it is important to remember the components of resentment and agressiveness which enter into the constellation of motivating forces. It is a special feature of successful suicide that we cannot afterwards explore with the child the reasons for its occurrence, and because of this limitation we cannot be sure that actual suicides arise from the same causes as attempted suicides and cases of purposive self-injury. Nevertheless these latter must be taken as danger signals, though the adults who are around the child should not become so alarmed as to subject him to a vigilance that will cripple his freedom.

Cases of suicide can almost be divided into two groups. Firstly, there is a very small number of really unhappy children who take their own lives and it usually is obvious afterwards that the adults around them were unaware of the severity of the child's sadness. This imposes on all of us who have responsibility for the care of children a challenge to be more perceptive than sometimes we are. Some authorities, however, consider that most child suicides occur 'out of the blue' in seemingly happy children, and if this were shown to be so it would follow that no amount of vigilance could prevent them.

The second group are usually teenagers whose relationships at home as well as among their coevals are unsatisfactory and who make suicidal attempts, mostly by taking sedative pills. Fortunately these generally recover and the task before the clinic is one of rehabilitation with parents and other nearly placed adults, so far as this can be achieved, and a therapeutic attempt to reduce resentments and to increase self-confidence and self-esteem. Two of our children who suffered from endogenous depression had attempted suicide by taking pills.

CHAPTER VI
Psychosomatic Illness and Emotion-linked Bodily States

In this group of conditions the problem does not present as anxiety or as disturbed behaviour but as a somatic symptom which ostensibly indicates disorder of function in the soma.[35] Only if the symptom is ignored – e.g. if the child is forced to go to school in spite of the abdominal pain – does free-floating anxiety emerge. There is, therefore, some justification for the contention that underlying anxiety, and often guilt and aggression as well, have been substituted externally by psychosomatic states. This is the old concept of the conversion symptom in hysteria, an idea which has been challenged in recent years.

Abdominal Pain
As do adults, children are wont to express their anxiety as a psychosomatic disorder and this most commonly takes the form of abdominal pain. These children are usually among the less difficult to treat. Obviously a physical examination is necessary to exclude the possibility of organic disease and if the family physician has not satisfied himself on this point either he or the psychiatrist may arrange for a pediatric consultation. The school doctor may perform this examination and there are some child psychiatrists who are prepared to do this themselves, but I always find it better to leave it to a colleague who is more regularly in touch with physical illness. One cannot afford to forget that these children are not immune from such complications as acute appendicitis or middle-ear infection.

Because of the episodic, recurrent nature of these pains someone has coined for them the term 'periodic syndrome', but it is doubtful wisdom thus to designate the symptom as though it were a specific disease.[36] Creak has noted the depressive, self-destructive element in these paroxysmal pains.[37] The attacks have occasionally been attributed to migraine and epilepsy has even been adduced as a rare cause.[38] It is better not to invoke such unusual possibilities unless there is evidence for their substantiation. Even then, while drugs might play a part in treatment regard would have to be paid to the fact that emotional factors influence migraine and even epilepsy. The pain often bears a time relationship to going to school and when this is so the right kind of parental support is quite important.

As regards treatment a small number of interviews involving superficial exploration of the child's circumstances, and reassurance, plus the appropriate contact, longer or shorter according to her needs, with the child's mother, will generally suffice. It is necessary to ensure that she understands the position and that she acquires reasonable confidence in supporting her child in the handling of his problem.

Headache and *vomiting* are among the commonest forms which psychosomatic illness may assume. Once the possibility of organic illness has been excluded it is important to discover psychological reasons for the symptom. In treatment the interplay of family relationships will usually be of paramount importance and enquiry should be made into what part the mother is playing, however unwittingly, as an ally of the child's unconscious motivation to be ill.

Anorexia nervosa is not particularly uncommon in teenage girls. Most take a severe form and require hospital treatment. Chloropromazine (largactil) in considerable dosage, with insistence on remaining in bed and temporary separation from parents, is the therapy of choice. Psychotherapy is delayed until the weight is nearly normal.[39]

Some girls make a response to out-patient treatment and I have recently treated a boy in regular weekly sessions over a period of some months. Lizzie had an I.Q. of 137 and had just left school with an encouraging number of 'O' level passes when her doctor referred her because she was taking slimming tablets. She had never been overweight, her mother considered her to be perceptibly thinner than her normal, but she would not eat anything containing flour or sugar. She had secondary amenorrhoea. Her father had been killed in the war when she was a baby, her mother had remarried some years later and there were now two younger children.

Lizzie had a somewhat rigid personality; she was fond of routine and she had not joined any of the school societies. We were unable to see her on more than one occasion on account of her reluctance to attend and on the second occasion her mother and stepfather came alone. Lizzie was keen to work on the land; arrangements had already been made for her to have a holiday with relatives and thereafter to take an agricultural course in a country area. With these plans we were in concurrence and we made an offer to see her again as occasion offered, should she be willing. Nine months later the family doctor wrote to say that Lizzie seemed well and was now a secret eater and that hidden condensed milk had been discovered where the slimming pills had earlier been found.

Our social worker called six and a half years after we had seen Lizzie. She was now teaching science in another part of the country and was enjoying her work. She remained thin, was faddy about food and avoided carbohydrate; she did not mix readily but engaged enthusiastically in a sporting activity with an older man whom she seemed to have adopted in some sense as a father figure. When she was home on holiday she was pleasant, but showed little warmth. It was not possible to adduce positively the cause of this girl's emotional illness, but it seems justifiable to conclude that she felt deprived and rejected, and as a result unworthy, on account of her father's death. To that extent she is one of a small number of children whom we have seen and whose problems stemmed from the circumstances of war.

Asthma, from the psychological standpoint, is ultimately a symptom of anxiety. The therapy of this serious disorder is an intimidating proposition. It is absolutely important to be wedded to the idea that the condition is psychologically motivated, but there are the strongest reasons for adhering also to the view that an underlying constitutional tendency exists. The evidence for this latter is first that only a small proportion of children (or adults) develop asthmatic attacks as a result of emotional stress, while the great majority of the population do not; and secondly the connection between asthma and *eczema*, which is so striking especially in those cases where the one condition alternates with the other.

Arnold, an intelligent boy of three and a half, was referred because of asthma which had developed six months previously. His parents, so far as we ever knew, were happily married and Arnold had been a wanted baby. His birth was three weeks premature, he was breast-fed for five months and was easily weaned from the bottle at nine months. He was never a contented baby, he cried a great deal, he did not sleep well in the first year of his life and he suffered a good deal from diarrhoea. He had never been a good eater and he often was tired, saying: 'I want to rest. My legs are hurting.'

Arnold was the middle of three boys and his older brother bullied him, would kick, punch or push him on the sly, took things from him and shouted at him. Similarly Arnold was jealous of his baby brother, pinching and biting him. To his mother he said 'I don't know why, I just wanted to bite him.' Arnold was a relatively solitary child. In subsequent treatment he showed much evidence of fearing to lose his mother and we felt that this, associated with the sibling rivalries, were among the causes of the insecurity and aggression which gave rise to the asthma. The reasons for his babyhood difficulties did not become clear to us and we may be justified in assuming that he was constitutionally less well endowed than some with the ability to withstand the ordinary stresses which any baby must meet at the beginning of life.

Balint[40] says that the child who has asthma is 'the presenting symptom of the mother'. Elsie was referred to us at the age of eight with a history of asthma since the age of eighteen months. An only child, she was an inhibited, shut-in little girl who made relationships with difficulty, looked younger than her years and lacked in attractiveness. She had attacks of asthma almost every night, but had been virtually free from them during two weeks when she was in hospital. Her mother was a complex-motivated individual whose emotions were repressed. She was beautiful, superficial and clever and she obviously dominated her little girl. It occurred one day that our psychologist visited a tea-room where Elsie's mother happened to be with several other ladies, and she was able to observe her, unknown to the mother. The way in which she had to be the centre of attraction and to dominate the conversation was impressive. The pediatrician, at an out-patient attendance soon after the asthma had been temporarily cured during the child's stay in hospital, remarked in his notes on how obviously pleased Elsie's mother had been to be able to tell him that the attacks had returned. The psychiatrist suspected that mother 'needed' Elsie's illness to justify her own claim for sympathy or praise.

Her father was more a background figure and a curious feature was that he had had an attack of asthma the year before Elsie came to see us. He seemed to have more time for Elsie than her mother had, but unfortunately he was away working in another part of the country and was home only at week-ends.

The asthma was considered to be due to emotional rejection, largely unconscious, on the mother's part, and the psychiatrist decided to take the mother in a series of therapeutic interviews. Her resistance, however, to this form of therapy was very strong and it was not possible to penetrate her defences. Elsie was then taken for treatment, but this was suspended after some weeks on account of the dubious prospects, and when a residential school for asthmatic children was recommended mother declined to accept this.

Five years after we first saw Elsie a letter of enquiry to her doctor received a reply in which he stated that her asthma was still a difficult problem, that she was going to boarding school, where her asthma was better, but that it was worse during the school holidays, and that with minimal doses of cortico-steroids she remained fairly well.

Elsie's asthma had had six and a half years in which to entrench itself before she came to the child guidance clinic. It is vitally important in the treatment of asthma that children should be brought to the clinic early in the course of the illness.

So far as the child's own unconscious motivation is concerned we may expect to find that anxiety and resentment are significant. Fear, either of punishment or of the overwhelming force of the emotions themselves, prevents their expression and ensures that they are largely excluded from consciousness. Our effort in therapy will be to put the child at ease and to enable him to express himself somehow, in the sand tray, in painting or in play with dolls. Freedom of expression is to be encouraged in play which is quite undirected by the therapist, but where the therapist is prepared to be stimulatingly helpful by suggesting that the child might try this or that. The child may be anxious to use the therapist, to get him to do certain things or to take part in certain forms of play, and the therapist will be inclined to follow the child's lead in this, however unsatisfactory this play may seem to be as a projection technique. Insight is, of course, essential, in the first place on the part of the therapist, who must find some meaning in the child's behaviour and attitudes. Once a relationship has been made and the child begins to trust the therapist as a friendly authority – for he is, after all, inevitably in that class of adults who are authorities – with whom he may risk taking a little liberty, he may begin to accept these interpretations and to add his own expressive comments.

A good deal of attention has been paid in the medical literature in recent years to hypnosis as a treatment for asthma. Clearly there are many problems in asthma which hypnosis will not solve, but where the illness is severe or other treatments are proving inadequate, it would seem less than justice not to invoke the help of a colleague expert in hypnotic techniques, if his intervention were likely to be of value. If in doubt, a conference with the hypnotist would enable a decision to be taken. Where other remedies have failed, or are likely to fail, serious thought should be given to residential schooling for a longer or shorter period. Some schools specialize in the treatment of asthma, but there may equally be a case for the residential school for maladjusted children with its umbrella of psychiatrically orientated child care. The treatment of asthma is a field which we share with the pediatrician and patients cannot but benefit from a cordial spirit of co-operation between us.

Recent experience is leading me to the view that there is, in these difficult cases of asthma, sometimes a case for the treatment of the parent rather than of the child. In one such case a girl was referred who had had various treatments elsewhere and it looked as though

PSYCHOSOMATIC ILLNESS

residential placement would be essential. It was only on seeing her father that I could appreciate that it was he who was in the more urgent need of therapy, and once his treatment was under way the girl's asthma ceased to be a problem.

Enuresis is a symptom regarding the etiology of which there are several theories, but no complete agreement. Kanner[41] says that the association of other features of anxiety and insecurity has been usual. Stalker and Band[42] found evidence of lack of cerebral inhibition as well as emotional trauma. Jones and Tibbetts[43] emphasized psychological causes, but discussed other theories of neuro-physiological anomaly. Soddy[44] states that enuresis is generally due to an emotional reaction, apart from rare congenital physical anomalies and slightly less rare neurological disorders. My own findings have led me to feel that, whatever other factors may be involved, continuing enuresis means that there is somewhere in the psyche a strong desire to remain a baby. Barbour and his colleagues found that no single causal factor accounted for enuresis, and they decided that it was reasonable to regard it as a delayed development or loss of bladder control which might be affected by many factors, physical and psychological.[45]

Bed-wetting which clears up for a week or two at a time and recurs, or which has been absent until some emotionally stressful episode such as the birth of a little brother, arises, or which remits during a stay in hospital only to recur on return home, can hardly have arisen from a failure of development. I saw a little girl who became dry when her mother was in hospital for a confinement, but started to wet after she came home: she also had an emotional swallowing difficulty which cleared up. A seven-year-old was off school with ear trouble for a week and was dry all the time, but wet his bed the night before going back to school. It looks as though bed-wetting were the safety valve for some emotional problem and perhaps it is a necessary symptom for some children at certain stages of their development. I believe that, without good evidence of other cause, we should, for practical purposes, regard enuresis as being ultimately dependent upon emotional factors. The following is one of the cases which are exceptions.

I was asked to see a girl of sixteen in the out-patients department of a general hospital. The complaint was occasional wetting by day, which was a matter of distress to her. She already had been referred to a gynaecologist, who had performed elaborate investigations including cystoscopy, and to a neurologist who found no abnormality, but who said there was just a possibility that the psychiatrist might discover something. I obtained from the girl the information that it was usually when she laughed that she wet herself, and afterwards her mother, who had come with her, asked to speak to me, saying that she had been refused permission to talk to either of the other specialists. She produced the interesting story that the girl had had a number of epileptic fits a year or two back. An E.E.G. was confirmatory and we had thus in the end considerable evidence of cerebral instability on which to base our treatment.

Remarks made by the mother of a nine-year-old boy who had been referred by a school medical officer to the clinic, in order to see if we could help clear up his bed-wetting, appeared to highlight the sort of emotional climate that is sometimes a part of our problem in dealing with such cases. Because the boy was insecure and anxious I offered to take him for weekly treatment, but I got the impression that his mother was dissatisfied because we did not recommend the electric bell. As they were leaving the building she was heard to remark: 'All that for nothing.' During my interview with her I had asked why it was that they had only one child and to this she had replied: 'One is enough to keep. . . .' The boy attended the clinic only a few times, after which his mother told the social worker that he appeared to be better, because he wet the bed less frequently when he was *not* coming to see me. We can hardly expect good results where a social atmosphere of this kind prevails.

In a different category was a mother who brought three of her children to the clinic because they wet their beds. Their ages varied from nine to six. There was a history of bed-wetting on the father's part and on the part of some of his relatives, the children themselves appeared average intellectually and the family seemed to be a warm, unaggressive group in which traces of insecurity lent attractiveness to the mother's personality and might also have some bearing on the bed-wetting. A younger child, aged three, had mild breath-holding attacks and she had had an operation for pyloric stenosis[46] at the age of four days.

Pituitary snuff, the electric bell and other measures had already been tried, and the mother found the triple problem burdensome. The treatment adopted was one of reassurance to her, in particular that she should not worry about the risk of bed-wetting persisting into adult life. Thirteen months later she told us that things were considerably better.

During my first term as a house physician at the Victoria Infirmary in Glasgow the ward sister asked me to try to do something to stop a boy patient wetting the bed. I could not remember as a student having received instruction in how to treat this disability – could medical schools pay more attention to everyday matters of this kind? - and I therefore consulted the drug list in the diary considerately provided by one of the well-known manufacturers and selected therefrom what seemed the most promising of the remedies listed. From that time onwards the boy had a dry bed. Such is the fickle nature of this complaint that I have never been so easily successful since.

A variety of drugs have a number of credits to their name. Ephedrine, gr. ½ to gr. 1, nocte, has sometimes proved useful. Disipidin, or pituitary snuff, one capsule insufflated nasally at bedtime, can be employed, using the insufflator supplied by the makers, and has had a number of authenticated successes. Burnett,[47] as a result of a chance observation, has suggested that 'preludin', because of its action on the hypothalamus, may be useful. Hypnosis has been recommended and has its quota of successes, but Rogers[48] gave an illustrative case to show that: 'When suggestion or persuasion cuts definitely across the deeper emotional purposes and needs, it can hardly be effective.' Paulett and Tuckman[49] outline a method which comes nearer to the core of the problem. Dealing with 'onset' enuresis – enuresis which has commenced after a period of being dry – they say: 'The mothers who came . . . for advice were given interviews at which they discussed with the doctor the problem of the onset enuresis in their children. . . . The children were not seen.' The authors do not seem to regard this form of therapy so efficacious for children who have never been dry. My personal experience also suggests that there are times when it is more practical to leave the child and to concentrate on his parents.

In the last year or two wide claims have been made for tofranil (imipramine), which one survey proved to have been much more effective than a placebo.[50]

The remaining form of physical treatment is the use of the *electric bell apparatus*. Reid[51] gave a stimulating account of the use of this equipment. He regards it as essential that the practitioner should fit up the apparatus in the child's bed and explain fully its working to the parent. He considers it necessary to wait until rapport with the child has been gained, when a short talk on enuresis can be given and the subject discussed with the parents. He then gives a sheet of general instructions to which he has added one or two points relevant specifically to this particular child. He has found a weekly home visit to be desirable in order to supervise the working of the machine and to assess the child's progress. He is prepared to use the bell from the age of five years. Thus the use of this instrument is not to be taken lightly, but its employment should be accompanied by serious attention to the principles, both mechanical and psychological, which are involved. It does, however, appear that the machine, if used aright, is quite the most valuable of the physical measures available to us for the treatment of bed-wetting.

For the broad purpose of therapy, although we cannot make hard and fast divisions between one group of children concerned and another, it will be useful to have a broad classification. *Firstly*, there are those children who wet their beds, who are anxious, inhibited and unhappy in themselves and whose nervousness appears to stem largely from circumstances of domestic unhappiness, ill-treatment, rejection or marked inability of parents to be understanding. *Secondly*, there are children who display much the same symptoms of insecurity – timidity, reserve, inability to mix well with others and so on – but where investigation suggests that the home background is a good one. *Thirdly*, there are a number of children who come from reasonable homes, whose adjustment to life and to their playmates appears satisfactory, but who still wet their beds. Into this category there probably fall a larger proportion of the older bed-wetters; the bed-wetting is likely to be the *cause* of secondary anxiety and the girl or boy is probably most anxious to have something done about it. Classification has also been made of a group of children who have been bed-wetters without intermission from babyhood and a second group of 'onset' enuretic children. Personally I have not found the distinction here to be of much therapeutic value, except that the latter group are probably easier to treat – but this does not mean that the mothers of the former group are less concerned to find a cure.

Where we are dealing with a bad domestic situation it seems futile to attempt any direct attack on the enuresis until everything possible has been done to ameliorate the environment. It is not only marital unhappiness or parental harshness that we may have to deal with but an obsessionally anxious attitude on the part of the mother to the enuresis or some other form of mental or nervous illness in a parent may be the problem at issue. If the domestic problem can be dealt with, then either the enuresis may clear up or the mother may find that it is no longer a serious burden to her and that she is prepared to let nature take its time in bringing about a cure. In those instances where the domestic problem remains it becomes a matter of judgment how far the child should have direct help in handling his emotional difficulties, the bed-wetting being regarded as merely one of these. Where parental co-operation is minimal one may be able to do little to help in any direction, at least for the time being.

In order to help mothers who must cope with wet beds under conditions of limited space or poor washing facilities, a colleague has devised a system whereby the clinic has a small supply of plastic mattress covers which can be loaned to the mothers.

In the second group, where we have a nervous child but where home circumstances are fair, the enuresis cannot usually be regarded as being the feature of greatest importance. Once the child's more general anxieties or personality difficulties have been dealt with as far as is reasonably practicable, then, if the enuresis remains, more specific attention can be devoted to this sympton.

Our third group – those in whom enuresis continues in the absence of other marked signs of maladjustment – will include those cases from the first two groups who continue to wet their beds after a satisfactory measure of adjustment has been achieved in other respects and we are, therefore, left with the problem of how to treat enuresis as such.

Having seen the child and made a rough assessment of his personality, reactions and intelligence, one then sees his mother in an attempt to judge what is her situation. If it is she, rather than the child, who needs help, we may leave the child with a word of encouragement. We can then make the attempt in one or two interviews with his mother – and perhaps once with father – to deal with her anxieties, guilt feelings, resentments and disappointments. The use of a chart on which the boy or girl lists wet and dry nights may stimulate a desire for success and assist in producing a co-operative effort between mother and child.

By virtue of the fact that many cases clear up with reassurance and the help of a drug, it is sound policy to begin by adopting an encouraging, supporting rôle. It will usually be wise to enhance the effect of this by prescribing, and pituitary snuff, ephedrine and tofranil all have their advocates. The doctor must himself be confident that the technique he is adopting has a reasonable chance of success. The confidence which the doctor's attitude imparts – it may be not so much the things he says but the way he says them and the manner in which he allies himself with the child – will be a considerable factor in making for success. We should not promise success where we cannot guarantee it, however, because failure would weaken our case when adopting any other, subsequent treatment.

If these relatively simple measures fail, does analytically orientated psychotherapy or play therapy hold out reasonable prospects? It has been my experience that often enough it has been possible in this way to achieve in the child a degree of self-confidence and a measure of better adjustment to his circumstances, but that the enuresis remains. What this probably means is that the level of emotional security achieved in the child and the level of emotional co-operation of which the parents have been made capable are still insufficient to break through the enuretic habit. The child is not yet quite ready to give up the emotional support which the symptom is providing.

The group of children, five-, six-, seven- or eight-year-olds or even more than this, who have never since birth been consistently dry, are a special case in point here. They are sometimes too insecure or too self-conscious about their contacts with adults to make a strong relationship in therapy. The way in which the anxieties of parents operate may profitably be considered further at this point. Why is it that a child whose bed is regularly wet at home is dry during a stay in hospital or that the matron of a children's home can achieve good results? Admittedly in the latter case the personality of the individual matron is important, but neither she nor the hospital nurses are subject to the influences of unconscious guilt, resentment, ambition or fear in relation to the child's development in the way that the mother is. For these reasons – the child's anxieties and, on the mother's part, emotional responses which it is not possible to eradicate – it will have to be accepted that there are many cases in which continued psychotherapy (or play therapy) is inappropriate as a treatment for enuresis.

In the event that suggestive therapy with the enhancement of drug medication has failed and psychotherapy is unsuitable or has already played its part in dealing with symptoms more amenable to its influence, we are left with the need of a further agent. It is here that the electric-bell apparatus comes into its own.

Encopresis – the German form of the word was introduced by Weissenberg in 1926 and was afterwards taken over into English by Charles Burns of Birmingham – means habitual soiling of the pants and sometimes of the bedclothes with faeces. From the mother's point of view it is a particularly annoying or even infuriating symptom and it has more of a social stigma than have most other kinds of childhood neurosis. These feelings are sometimes enhanced by the circumstance that the child appears to be doing it deliberately. One mother described how her son obviously enjoyed defecating in his trousers, standing in the corner of the room to do so. We have also on occasion met the child who could desist from the habit for as long as a week in order to obtain some concession from his parents and who would, thereafter, revert to soiling. In addition, there are those children who defecate in inappropriate parts of the house, hide faeces behind furniture or smear it on the wall and in one case even on the ceiling. We may also include those little children who refuse to defecate for days on end and who thus cause their mothers considerable anxiety because, although this is not regarded as encopresis, it is a symptom of a more fundamental nature and its study may teach us something of the underlying nature of the disorder which displays itself as soiling in older children.

The baby or toddler who refuses to defecate may be frankly afraid. He may already have hurt himself in some way while on the potty or he may be terrified of losing this piece of himself. A great deal of maternal patience as well as comprehension will be called for in helping the child to overcome these real apprehensions, and it may be the child psychiatrist's task to assist her in doing so, or even in direct therapy with the child to unearth and to allay these fears. We already have seen how constipation[52] may be a reaction to emotional stress and the relationship between anxiety and diarrhoea is well known.

Anthony[53] divided encopretic children into three categories. First there are those who have never been clean, whom he regarded as coming from unsatisfactory families, and who did not require psychotherapy but should have habit training for a few months under happier conditions. This form he called 'continuous'. The second, or 'discontinuous', type occurs in compulsively motivated children whose mothers are meticulously clean and have applied rigid toilet training. The children are inhibited and require prolonged psychotherapy. The third category is that of 'retentive' encopresis in which an obsessive mother has enforced severe toilet training and the child has reacted with stubborn constipation. Here again therapy will be called for with emphasis on maternal ability to co-operate. These concepts provide valuable guide lines to therapy.

A Birmingham survey, unpublished, in which I co-operated, showed a wide distribution throughout the intelligence scale and a high proportion of anxious, inhibited, insecure or timid children. A further one-fifth had tagged on to them one or other of the adjectives, 'aggressive', 'moody', 'stubborn', 'resentful', 'highly strung' and 'spoilt'. Enuresis was a part of the symptom complex in more than half of the eighty cases which were adequately documented. Schooling did not appear to be a significant stress. A large majority were boys, a finding which matches those of other surveys.

Woodmansey[54] has produced strong evidence to show that the main, although not the only, cause of constipation and of soiling is toilet training and that treatment will generally involve 'un-training'. This process of un-training is calculated to produce a state of affairs in which the child, freed from all threat of disapproval, is at liberty to defecate as and when he feels and thus to develop naturally himself those habits which are socially advantageous.

It is a good clinical rule that physical examination should precede therapy, mainly with a view to discovering and dealing with those children who are severely constipated, and it is my own practice to rely upon the services of the pediatrician or the general practitioner for this purpose.

The above observations notwithstanding, a clinical appraisal of cases compels the view that we are left with a child who is emotionally maladjusted, who has a deep sense of rejection, who carries a heavy load of unconscious guilt and in whose motivation hidden resentments frequently play a part. The uninitiated are inclined to believe that the encopretic child becomes aware, just like everyone else, that faeces require to pass, but that for some reason he does not or cannot hold them back until the appropriate moment. But from questioning some children and from an appraisal of attitudes in others, I am convinced that this is not so, but that the child becomes aware only when faeces are actually passing through the anus, or has actually been voided. There may be exceptions to this – we have mentioned the child who was able to hold her encopretic function in abeyance for days in order to obtain parental concessions – but this unawareness until too late must be regarded as a usual feature of psychological soiling.

Treatment must pay regard to the personalities of parents and particularly of the mother, who is usually the person who has dealt with toilet training in babyhood and who is most affected by the continued soiling. Often she will need not only support but a better understanding of her own motivation. We have seen a number of cases where parental attitudes, unconscious in their motivation, contribute to the problem, and in some cases there has been a kind of connivance with the child in his unwillingness to take the necessary steps to overcome the habit. One mother of a four-year-old boy suffered from a strong sense of inferiority and the treatment consisted in a short series of psychotherapic interviews with her coupled with some adjustment of the domestic arrangements. The soiling ceased. It recommenced, however, about six weeks later, but the therapist was not told of this nor was he again consulted until the boy had been encopretic for a number of years. In the meantime he had been taken to a pediatrician, and in the event various remedies, including finally a couple of terms at a residential school for younger maladjusted children, were necessary to produce a cure. What emotional resistance on the part of this young woman, who had responded well to her own treatment and who had gained a cessation of the child's symptom, prevented her earlier return, never became clear. A mother who brought her little boy at the age of three because of his refusal to use the potty and his insistence on defecating into his clothes, had herself had a series of sessions with a marriage counsellor on account of her frigidity. The frigidity persisted and it seemed unlikely that it would respond to treatment, wherefore it was decided that the child should come for play therapy in the clinic. After about three sessions the mother began to make excuses why she could not bring him, such as a telephone call we had from her husband to say that she did not feel well, but after two or three further weeks she just stopped and there were no further phone calls or letters. The coexistence of the mother's genital frigidity and her little boy's anal 'frigidity' invites speculation.

If therapy with children who are encopretic is to prosper it must be in an atmosphere of liaison with a child who is motivated to discard the symptom and who manages to have confidence in the therapist's desire genuinely to be helpful. If the symptom is ensuring that the child can remain a baby, cut off from other children who ostracize him because of the encopresis, enjoying his mother's full attention and controlling her actions, and if he is not yet ready to give up these fantasies, then he can hardly be expected to co-operate in a programme of treatment.

The type of case we have found most difficult to treat is that of the child who has strong guilt feelings. The encopresis, which he is unconsciously motivated to commit is frowned upon by parental authority. It is the story over again of the baby who derives pleasure from evacuation and messing, but whose mother stresses habit training, thus producing a serious emotional conflict between desire and guilt. Although such a situation in babyhood may be the cause of soiling later on, it would be far too great a simplification to suggest that it is the main cause of the difficult type of case we are now considering, because in the meantime elements of sexual guilt have added themselves to the anal erotic position and the severe anxieties involved are overlaid by powerful defences. To break these down can be quite difficult. The therapist who implies that the erotic impulses are not, after all, so wicked, is visualized as allied to the devil and is therefore dangerous to the unstable state of mental equilibrium at which the child's emotional processes have arrived and which the child, unconsciously, sees as the only alternative to emotional chaos. In this dilemma it may be of some help to give to the child the interpretation that he is, in fact, feeling that the therapist is being bad, or 'rude', which is the word that our Midland children seem to employ when talking to their parents, and to say to the child that of course he feels a bit frightened because the therapist is behaving in this way. The therapist may then go on to explain that sex cannot really be so bad, since it is Nature's, or God's, way of bringing new life into the world. Occasionally, at the end of such an interview I have said to the mother, in the child's presence, that we have been talking of these things.

TREATMENT FOR CHILDREN

In these more difficult cases one aims to achieve a good therapeutic relationship in which the child's reactions, elicited through play or painting, can be discussed; but so limited will one's success in this direction sometimes turn out to be that we cannot afford to leave any stone unturned in the area of parental and sibling relationships nor in the field of the child's wider social contacts. In such an atmosphere of therapeutic co-operation success is attainable, but may take time. Residential treatment is not a course which one would naturally expect to be helpful in a condition in which insecurity and guilt are so prominent factors. Exceptionally, however, where child-parent relationships are characterized by a high degree of mutual interdependence and where the unconscious stresses on both sides are impossible to resolve, we may be able to get both the child and his parents to agree to residential care for a time, and in such instances it can achieve satisfactory results.

Tics are a common manifestation of anxiety, although there is some evidence that antenatal factors in the mother's health and neonatal weakness on the child's part are influential.[55] The temptation to prescribe drugs should be resisted, as these are not helpful. The probable influence of emotional conflict at home has to be borne in mind as well as the need for a forbearing, sympathetic and optimistic attitude on the part of mother, and father, too. The child's mother may expect that the therapist should cure the tic, whereas the therapist will ask for a positive contribution from her. Caution, rather than optimism, is a wise approach. The anxieties of parents, which underlie the attitudes which they display, call for help.

In treatment it is not the easiest of things to get the confidence of these children, who are apt to be at pains to hide the nature of the nuclear anxieties which underlie the symptom and which involve feelings of unworthiness that are too painful to tolerate in consciousness. It is as well to aim at a short, rather intensive treatment, involving both child and his mother, and not forgetting his father's influence.

Often it will be better to treat mother rather than child. The great need for the child is that his parents should accept him as he is, tic and all, and love him uncritically. Exhortation to desist from the tic is simply a form of rejection and is detrimental. It is the mother's own unconscious feelings of guilt and failure that are the force behind the pressure she exerts. This will not always be the situation in cases of tic, but where it is the need will be to help the mother to unravel the complexes that are causing her to feel guilty, to need to have a child who is perfect, to be overanxious about his future, to identify with him and worry because he is teased at school or to wonder where she has failed her child or her husband in being in some way responsible for the tic. A gulf tends to appear between the child who has an annoying symptom and the parent who cannot resist the temptation to nag and by analysing the mother's feelings we may enable this gulf to be bridged. If father is impatient of the symptom he may, unwittingly, be imposing a strain on both mother and child, and it will help if we can instil some insight into what is happening in himself and what may be its effect on other members of the family.

A particularly awkward form is the verbal or swearing tic which has been given the special designation of *'Gilles de la Tourette's* syndrome'. Bockner[56] says that the onset usually occurs in childhood and that tics are followed by compulsive sounds and these by obscene words. These children have a sombre prognosis and this is one of the few conditions in child psychiatry where major reliance will have to be placed on a tranquillizing drug such as chlorpromazine or haloperidol.[57]

Corbett *et al.*, in a recent survey of 180 *'tiqueurs'*, found that two-thirds of all those followed up for eight years or more were fully recovered from their tics, but there was an increased incidence of anxiety and depressive symptoms. The incidence of total recovery was identical between treated and untreated cases.[58] Yet we may still hope that the kind of family therapy outlined above will confer some benefit.

Colitis. In adult psychiatry, whatever organic factors may be regarded as underlying this condition, its psychological features are recognized as conversion ones, the diarrhoea being the exteriorization of unconscious anxiety and hostility. In child psychiatry one is reluctant to admit the existence of a developed state of conversion hysteria, but the psychosomatic nature of the illness will hardly be called in question. Soddy[59] points out how ulcerative colitis in a child can cause a crippling family anxiety and how the symptom and the family's anxieties can both fluctuate and be interwoven through a period of years. Woodmansey[60] has shown that ulcerative colitis arises from the circumstance that the patient is angry, but that there is fear of expressing the anger, so that the former is repressed and the colitis arises from the conflict in which the fear has overcome the need to express the anger.

Pica is the eating of earth, dust and such material, while *coprophagy* is the ingestion of faeces. Certainly the former and perhaps exceptionally the latter can be normal behaviour, occasionally in babies. Coprophagy is usually a symptom of more or less severe subnormality. If pica continues beyond babyhood it will call for positive attention and may warrant an intelligence assessment. It is said to be due sometimes to worms, malnutrition or anaemia, and this possibility is, therefore, worth considering. The emotional association between food and love may be relevant and the total relationship between child and parents, as well as others in the environment, is important. One would suspect that hidden away somewhere there is a want of closeness or a lack of adequate understanding between parents and child. It is probably this that needs to be unearthed.

Eczema must be regarded as an organic disorder of skin metabolism the psychological concomitants of which, though important, are secondary. Soddy[61] says that it can be a terrible scourge. He says it is very difficult for a mother to give herself whole-heartedly to the nursing of her eczematous baby, who may therefore be deprived of nursing warmth. Warin,[62] referring to his own and other studies on the prognosis of infantile eczema, says that mild cases have a satisfactory prognosis, although the severe ones are usually very persistent. The discovery of steroids in treatment has greatly improved the immediate prognosis. Phenobarbitone is not without value.

It will be wise to leave the treatment of eczema in the hands of the general practitioner and the pediatrician except in so far as the child guidance clinic is asked to deal with emotional aspects. Treatment will follow the lines of attention both to the child's anxieties and to those of the mother. The reactions of father and of siblings are important and we attempt to understand and to alleviate the emotional stresses which are operating within the family – some of these no doubt due to the child's illness, but others existing independently of it and aggravating it. By purposeful therapy along these lines we may reasonably hope to decrease the burden of unhappiness which the child and his mother are carrying and in many cases favourably to influence the child's chances of recovery from his eczema.

Urticaria is seldom a serious problem, but the following case is of such interest as to justify description. Three young children in a family with whom the writer was closely connected all suffered from urticaria. In the case of the eldest, this cleared up fairly soon, but the other two children suffered for several years from severe urticaria which never remitted completely and which often included large areas of skin, principally legs, abdomen and arms. No physical abnormalities were discovered, tests for allergy were considered positive for some foods and for some clothing, but thorough restriction in these respects produced no amelioration. Calamine lotion and dressings were the rule for years on end. There was no obvious psychiatric disturbance. O'Donovan, dermatologist to the London Hospital, was eventually consulted and suggested a month's course of luminal for both children. The younger child became sleepy with this and it was discontinued after a few days, but the elder had the full course. About a week after the luminal course was completed by the elder child the urticaria suddenly cleared up in *both* children, and never returned. Twenty years have passed since then. O'Donovan told of a similarly striking success he had had earlier in a child who was the son of an internationally famous politician. I can offer no positive explanation of these cures.

Migraine, although it must be regarded as having ultimately a constitutional or organic root, is often associated with emotional problems, and in adult cases we may expect to be able to achieve appreciable improvement by psychotherapy. The same should be true of children, though not many with true migraine are referred to the clinic. Inheritancewise there is some evidence of a connection between epilepsy and migraine. There seems also to be a connection with cyclical vomiting, in that the parents of a child who suffers from this complaint may themselves suffer from migraine, or the child may suffer from periodic headache or develop migraine later.

Patrick was thirteen when he came to see us. He was the elder of two boys, his I.Q. was 132 and he suffered from attacks of migraine in which his vision failed gradually, ending in blindness which lasted for a few seconds. He was also afraid of going upstairs, especially at night – 'I want to go, but something stops me' – he would cry or scream if rebuked at home, he was jealous of his brother who had a happier nature, and he had a difficult relationship with his mother. He did reasonably well at grammar school, but became upset over his homework. He had several hobbies, but soon lost interest in these; for a time he was in the Scouts and for a time a member of a club. With this latter group he had enjoyed climbing Snowdon by night, an interesting contrast to his fear of climbing the stair at home. He was subject to moods of depression and told me how, on some days, he awoke feeling unhappy. As a baby he was breast fed for three months, then bottle fed, but was frequently sick and there was difficulty in getting him to sleep. At the age of eight he was in hospital for a hernia operation and was very nervous after he came home. His home was a happy one and his parents, both of whom incidentally were members of the town council, naturally affectionate.

Patrick's treatment consisted of psychotherapy virtually all at a conscious level. He was seen on twenty-four occasions over a period of nearly a year. A relationship with the therapist within which his problems were discussed enabled him to achieve a degree of self-confidence. Almost seven years after he first came to us we had a letter from his mother in which she said Patrick was quite well, was an apprentice in the engineering trade and enjoyed this work.

CHAPTER VII

Problems Related to Education

School phobia, which is an anxiety-motivated refusal to attend school, is usually a symptom of fears of a deeper nature. The problem *appears* to have become greater in recent years and several workers have made literary contributions, notably Kahn, who has both reviewed the literature and written extensively about the subject himself.[63]

Some workers have said that school phobia is a separation anxiety on the part of the child, who is terrified to be away from his mother, but this is not the whole truth, as the child often will accept voluntary separations such as visits to relatives or to the swimming baths. It is the separation in an area which is controlled by authority and where demands are made upon the child to stand up for himself which seems to imperil his limited ego strength. Jung says: 'The neurotic who cannot leave his mother has good reasons; the fear of death holds him there. It seems as if no idea and no word were strong enough to express the meaning of this'.[64]

In a personal series of sixty-six cases[65] the level of intelligence played little part in determining the disability, but three-quarters of the children affected were boys and very nearly three-quarters were eleven years old or over, so that the problem appeared to be one mainly involving the secondary school. The reason for this was not clear.

The child withdraws into the family setting like a baby and in this limited sphere he enjoys a correspondingly limited measure of happiness, while in contrast to his timidity outside the home, *within* he sometimes is demanding and if he does not get his own way, aggressive. Underlying the condition there is probably an unconscious fear of the loss of his parents' love arising from oedipal stress, guilt and aggression towards parental figures having made him afraid of not being loved and, therefore, utterly dependent on continuing demonstrations of love. This results, too, in feelings of unworthiness and of being inferior to other boys. Frequently we find that the mother reinforces the boy's sense of dependence in not having taken responsibility for encouraging him to meet the normal obstacles of life. Instead she has allowed him to burrow back into the family and has herself unconsciously, if not openly, enjoyed his dependence and the resultant symbiotic relationship between them. It may be because a similarly unhealthy father-daughter relationship is seldom so strongly developed that school phobia is less common in girls. In my own series we were able to claim that in two-fifths of the number parental attitudes were a major cause of the school refusal. Just over one-third appeared to be suffering from potentially hysterical or phobic neurosis, usually without discoverable stress-producing background circumstances sufficient to account for the neurosis. A striking impression, clinically, is that these children have lost faith in themselves.

In approaching treatment one has first to assess the child and to make a decision as to whether or not he is emotionally fit to attend school, provided he can be given the necessary support. It then becomes a case of assessing the parents, and if there is a chance that they will be able to co-operate I point out to them how essential it is that they should take a firm line in insisting that the child should return, while themselves continuing to be understanding and sympathetic. I point out that they must be able to bear both the child's tears and his kicks beforehand without either becoming anxious or getting angry; knowing that the child cannot help this behaviour they will not be cross, but at the same time, because they place their faith in the doctor's judgment they will not be overanxious or upset.

Just how one puts this across to parents will depend a good deal on the idiosyncrasies of the individual doctor. I have said: 'If Jean were going to be so upset by your insistence that she goes back to school, that she would jump out of the upstairs window, then I should not suggest this; but I am sure that that will not happen.' Naturally, one has to be sure. In one case the mother had temporarily to give up work, while insisting on the child's return to school, on account of the latter's anxieties. Sometimes the parents, rather than the child, will need several interviews with the doctor.

The teacher's patient co-operation is also necessary, and in cases where the child is not fit for immediate, full return to school, some adjustment may, however, make this possible. This adjustment should be coupled with parental support for the child and perhaps reinforced by a small number of interviews in the clinic, or with the school doctor if it is she who is handling the case.

Hood has illustrated the importance of the earliest possible referral to the child guidance clinic of cases of school phobia and the giving of an immediate appointment once those children are referred. He then treats the child's problem analytically in a small number of interviews, seeks the full co-operation of the teacher and encourages the earliest possible return to school.[66]

It is in those cases where handling of the situation along such lines as the above would have been advised but where parents fall short that some quasi-legal remedy may have to be considered. For example, it may be obvious that we shall never get this boy or that girl back to school so long as he is under the influence, in the matter, of his anxious parents. In some such cases we have known these children, once admitted to a residential school for maladjusted children, to settle down there quickly and happily and to benefit immensely from the change. This usually needs the co-operation of the director of education and, from the parents, their formal consent. Who actually takes the child to the residential school is not unimportant, and if the parents cannot do so, it is likely that someone such as the social worker or the educational psychologist will be prepared to find the time to make the necessary journey. This is someone whom the child already knows and can trust.

For some children early return to school will not be possible and residential schooling will for one reason or another be inappropriate or not available. More or less lengthy treatment in the clinic may then be called for and this will not differ materially from play therapy or psychotherapy when given for any other symptom or illness. While return to school is then a very desirable goal, it may not be the main objective of treatment which is, rather, to fit the child for adequate living; and there will be a minimum number of cases where treatment can be regarded as having achieved much, even though the child never returned to school.

In one or two areas special provision is made for children who find attendance at ordinary school too much for them and in whose cases early return is seen to be unobtainable. One such is the Remedial Teaching Centre in West Bromwich. This may be regarded as a kindergarten school in so far as it concerns the school phobia children and it offers a useful, and not unduly expensive, form of treatment.

Not infrequently it happens that the child requests a change to a different school and that this request receives parental support. Only exceptionally has such a change, in my experience, been attended by success, but sometimes we have deemed it right to give it a trial so that, if it fails and we have to recommend residential school, we shall have a stronger hand in doing so.

The interpretation of a dream played an interesting part in the treatment of a thirteen-year-old boy. Everything was blue around; there was a white balloon filled with water and the patient was inside the balloon feeling very uncomfortable and a little afraid. He wanted to get through the outlet pipe, but each time he tried his shoulders caught. The obstetric symbolism of this dream is obvious, but its interpretation will depend to some extent on how far one accepts the possibility of unconscious memories reaching so far back in time. The alternative possibility is that knowledge acquired later of what happens at birth may be built into a dream. At all events the dream must represent his conflict – he is uncomfortable and afraid because he is still so dependent on his mother – he tries to break away from this dependence and yet he cannot (his shoulders are caught) and each time he is, so to speak, thrown back into his mother's arms. The therapist attempted to put this interpretation across, referring to his dependence on his mother and pointing out that somehow it must be more to his advantage to remain a little boy than to be a big boy – since this is what he is doing, it must somehow be to his advantage to do it – and Billy accepted this interpretation to the extent of saying that he felt guilty about Mum having to do so much for him, and it came out that he actually wanted her to be at school with him. What one is trying to do is to give insight to the patient so that he can grasp the meaning of the emotional problem that is within him.

A symbolic incident cropped up at the end of the interview in which this dream was discussed, although it was only afterwards that there became apparent to the therapist its meaning and the meaning of the part he had played in it. Billy's home was some way out of town and he had to come into town to visit the clinic. On this occasion he said to the therapist that he was having difficulty in finding his way about the town and the therapist, with a view as he consciously thought to encouraging the boy and building up the relationship between them, took him out to a bookseller and bought him a local map. What he afterwards realized was that Billy was really telling him that he was finding it difficult to find his way around in the big adult world into which he was trying to emerge and that he, the therapist, had (unconsciously) been giving him a map of life.

A girl of ten and a half years was referred, an attractive but not robust child of average intelligence. Both parents were of an anxious cast, but family relationships were good. The loss of a brother before her birth had created stresses from the effects of which she may have suffered. The child herself had feeding difficulties in infancy; her mother had 'milk fever', so that she never was breast fed and she had not taken well to the bottle. At the age of five she found the school situation stressful and developed alopecia. As regards etiology, we considered that even if there were not features of truly constitutional origin there were certainly qualities of family neurosis which, together with the girl's lack of robustness and her alopecia, would go a long way towards explaining the problem.

Treatment in the clinic was confined to a very few interviews, largely on account of the fact that the therapist was shortly leaving for an extended holiday, but before he left she was attending school, afternoons only, and her mother said that the child had been much happier. In the mornings her mother had to go out to work, so that the girl was often alone in the house. A few weeks later the therapist, remembering the tenuous nature of her attachment to school, sent her a postcard from Rhodesia. It arrived in the middle of the morning. She immediately wrote a note to her mother to say that she had gone to school, and from that day to this, which is many months afterwards, she has attended regularly, morning and afternoon, although often being late in the morning. She said this was not due to the receipt of the postcard, her mother said it was, and perhaps the distance from which the card had come gave it sufficient enchantment as an assurance that she was not uncared for, either within her family or outside.

Speech Difficulties. A large part of the province of speech disorder is outside child psychiatry and in practice child psychiatrists need usually concern themselves with only three types of speech problem, namely: children who do not speak or whose speech is delayed, children who lose their speech and children who stammer. Those who do not speak are usually cases of delayed speech and when an intelligence test is done many turn out to be backward. It is assumed that deafness and other possible organic factors have been excluded. Exceptionally emotional trauma may have prevented the child from speaking, and in either case support given to the parents is often the best therapy. Loss of speech may result from the emotional concomitants of some physical illness or from other emotional trauma or it may be an early symptom of psychosis. Often refusal to speak is selective, as in the case of Christine, aged six, I.Q. 107, who would not speak to teachers or to most boys and girls. Nor would she go to the lavatory at school or sit on the potty in front of her mother at home. She was described as a difficult, stubborn baby, did not say sentences till three or three and a half years and started to wet the bed after her brother, Philip, was born. She had some actual difficulty in pronouncing certain letters and she told her mother that she could not say 'Philip'. Her mother appeared to have an inhibited personality.

Because there was no improvement within a couple of months of Christine's coming to see us, we took her for treatment sessions with a view to making a relationship which might add to her self-confidence. Later on, her mother asked her teacher home to tea and Christine spoke freely to her. Two and a quarter years after we first saw her there was considerable improvement and she was said to be talking at school, and a further eighteen months afterwards she was described as greatly improved. A change to a private school with smaller classes played a part. Christine had a lively imagination and her treatment sessions consisted almost entirely of her imaginative play and of a relationship formation towards the therapist. In the end we were left with the impression that the passage of time, along with the adjustments that were made, may have played a larger part in bringing about the improvement than did the treatment.

Stammering is the major speech problem of child guidance. As a matter of practice the great majority of children who stammer are referred to the speech therapist; as a matter of experience speech therapists consider the treatment of stammering to be within their competence and it is a matter for reflection that they seem to do so without having the benefit of the psychologist's assessment or the social worker's help. How far speech therapists are justified in attempting to treat emotional disturbances is evidently a matter of some controversy, as was apparent from a correspondence which I instituted several years ago.[67] In the present state of the child health services of this country, however, there is a great deal to be said for fostering a spirit of co-operation between speech therapy and the child guidance clinics. The risk, as it appears to me, is that the speech therapists may insulate themselves in a defensive position because they fear to discover the limitations of their therapeutic competence, while some at least of child guidance clinics may claim an omniscience which is entirely illusory.

There still exists in informed circles a good deal of doubt and difference of opinion regarding the cause of stammer. When it occurs between the ages of two and four years it usually is physiological and can be disregarded. It is widely claimed that there must be a combination of causative factors of which the psychological is one, and it has been held that psychogenic symptoms, though frequent, may be mostly secondary to the stammer. Customarily a stammer disappears when the patient is angry, when he is alone or on the occasion of some verbal interjection, and it may disappear when he is hypnotized or as a result of sedative drugs – pointers which surely indicate a non-organic cause.

The literature on stammering has often reflected a clutching at this or that possible straw of causation and where treatment is concerned has been so indecisive that the student has every justification to think that we are merely groping when we try to treat this disability. Bonnard has quoted the case of a severe stammer in an eight-year-old boy, which was improved by one, and strikingly improved by eight psychiatric interviews in which its underlying meaning as an aggressive defence against fantasied punishment had been conveyed to him.[68]

TREATMENT FOR CHILDREN

Barbara has stressed the necessity to treat the entire personality and has drawn attention to the need for co-operation between speech therapist and psychotherapist.[69] Attention to the mother's and father's attitudes – especially their anxieties towards their child and the aggressions his symptom arouses within them – are often no less important than any direct therapy given to the child. Repressed anxiety and repressed aggression seem to be the usual causes of stammer. Possibly the aggressive element is the reason why the disorder is commoner in boys than in girls. A little boy who was referred to us was the elder of two brothers. On the occasion of a visit from relatives the younger was given a great deal of praise and attention and a better present was handed to him. The following morning the older child commenced to stammer and the stammer persisted. One is reminded here of William Moodie's dictum: 'Incidents do not cause neurosis; influences do.' Such influences must have been at work in this boy's environment long before the visit of the relatives. Kanner points out that stammer afflicts people of nearly every class among, at any rate, the advanced races, and that it is rare or unknown in diabetics. He quotes Hill as saying that it occurs when the individual cannot immediately adjust to urgent circumstances.

Worster-Drought has stated that few cases in his experience are relieved of their stammer by psychotherapeutic, or even psychoanalytical methods alone. My own experience has been that cases of established stammer are usually impossible to cure. The emotions that are repressed are (unconsciously) felt to be so dangerous and the (unconscious) fear of punishment for entertaining them is so great that the defence against the emergence of insight is impregnable. The only system which appears at the present time to offer much prospect in the treatment of stammer on a large scale is that it should be treated early and that, with this object in view, children should be referred to the child guidance clinic as soon as the condition appears to persist.

The anxious parent exerts emotional pressure on the child, albeit unwittingly. This anxiety needs to be replaced by an ability to enjoy the child for himself, and as he is. In treating the child we must attempt to discover what is his nuclear problem and endeavour to get across to him an understanding of what this is. Unless a treatment policy of this nature gives promise of improvement within a reasonably short time it is purposeless to persist indefinitely. The best answer to the problem which stammering presents would be a larger number of analytically trained child therapists.

The case of a boy who was taken for treatment, at the request of the speech therapist, but also as an experiment to test the above-mentioned theory, will illustrate the difficulties. The therapist used every manoeuvre to get expression of feelings, but, except for the expression at an intellectual level of such things as minor resentments against school prefects, nothing was forthcoming. Paintings had added nothing to what we already knew or were able to talk about, and at this juncture the therapist asked the patient to make a scene in the sand tray.

The result was interesting, namely a massacre (his own word for it), and that was what it looked like – a fence across the middle of the ground, machine guns on one side and numerous dead and wounded lying in the sand on the other side. He said it would give him a kind of savage pleasure, and most people, he thought, would feel the same, to see a film where machine guns mowed down the enemy in the nick of time, just saving British troops from annihilation. Here was clear evidence of aggression and reason to hope that insight could be achieved. Intellectually the boy could see the point, but beyond this we could not get and he could not emotionally grasp his hatreds, resentments or jealousies. After two or three further interviews in which the therapist twisted and turned every way possible in the hope of bringing these emotions into consciousness, but without avail, he decided to discontinue treatment. This termination was effected amicably, the therapist feeling however, that the patient took the therapist's decision very blandly. He made the suggestion that if the problem were still causing the patient concern after he reached the age of eighteen, it might be worth while to consider further therapy.

Three years after this boy's last interview in our clinic we heard, on reliable information from a professional colleague, that the stammer was much worse and that he had been referred to one of the psychiatrists at a local mental hospital. Neither this psychiatrist nor the family doctor made any enquiry regarding his earlier treatment at the child guidance clinic.

To adopt an attitude of befogged optimism in the face of realities is unlikely to do much service to our patients. Surely it is better to recognize the limitations of therapeutic possibility and to aim for targets which assessment of the circumstances suggests as being realizable.

A second boy, whose situation was similar, was also taken for treatment and the result appeared equally unpromising. Yet he returned to see us two or three years afterwards, this time in order to discuss his future career; and when the therapist remarked on the evident improvement in his speech, he replied that some of the things which he had discovered during his psychotherapy had proved valuable.

The Americans seem to prefer the word 'stutter', rather than 'stammer', but the terms are synonymous.

TREATMENT FOR CHILDREN

We were asked to see a boy of fourteen and a half years who had already had a considerable period of speech therapy for his stammer, which, however, was persisting. His intelligence quotient turned out to be 90, and the psychologist noted that he stammered in the test situation, but not when making spontaneous conversation. He had one older and one younger sister, both of whom were attractive and were considered to be brighter than he. At one time his father had left his mother and both had 'messed around' with other partners, but they had come together again. His mother adopted an overprotective attitude towards the boy. He himself was quiet, polite and inhibited. He stammered often, but his speech otherwise was clear. It was interesting that his father, who was inclined to strictness with him, had himself stammered until he was sixteen. At school the boy was badly teased, and his headmaster said he could shout and swear in the playground.

It was decided that he should continue in speech therapy, which he did. When, seven years and nine months later, our social worker visited his home in connection with a survey we were conducting, his mother said that the stammer was no longer a hardship and that it occurred only when he was excited or anxious. He had by this time had one year at technical college and had served a five-year apprenticeship, had numerous friends and had his own car. She spoke warmly of the benefit he had received from speech therapy. It is probable that many of our cases of stammering achieve this sort of intermediately good result, and in this imperfect world it is a truism that half a loaf is better than no bread.

Reading disability, dyslexia or word blindness, is another condition where disparity exists between those who hold an emotional view and those who regard organic factors as being the major cause. Some cases, of course, are due to demonstrable organic illness, traumatic, infective or vascular, but this is not to say that reading disability in an otherwise healthy child is necessarily organic in origin. Bower considers that there must be some cerebral disturbance of a reversal or a symbolic kind, and Hallgren has established that the condition is transmitted genetically,[70] while Hermann has made out a strong case for a familial incidence of 'congenital word blindness' or 'specific dyslexia'.[71] He says that it occurs to some degree in 10 per cent of the population and that the great majority of backward readers in schools are suffering from this. On the other hand, psychoanalysis has shown that in some cases inability to learn to read is due to guilt, whereby the acquiring of sexual knowledge is forbidden (at an unconscious level) and that this emotional inhibition extends then to all knowledge.

EDUCATIONAL STRESS

We were asked to see Miriam because she could not learn to read well. She was eleven years old and both her parents and her teachers regarded her as immature. She had two younger sisters, the older of whom was almost nine and who could read better than she. Her father was a bank clerk and the family appeared to jog along pretty well together, but we came to regard the mother as neurotic, anxious, without insight and unable to enjoy her children. Miriam's non-verbal I.Q. was 125, but her verbal was only 114. She had, however, an over-all scatter of from 94 to 149. She was good at arithmetic. (Psychoanalysis has revealed that some girls dislike long division because of the down-straggling contour of the sum, which suggests the penis and arouses unconscious penis envy.)[72] She said she hated school, Miss Browne was horrible and some children had stolen £15 worth of goods.

In a session which was typical of Miriam's response the therapist asked what she would like to do. Miriam did not know and she just sat in the chair looking at him. The therapist commented that there was something in Miriam that did not allow her to do what she wanted and that he wondered what she would do if she felt free to do just whatever she liked. For example, she might even feel like doing something to him. Miriam said that she liked to tidy things! The therapist said that this amounted to getting everything straight and correct and Miriam said, 'Yes.' She said she liked modelling and the therapist suggested having some water in the sand tray, but even when he gave her the water tin she had to ask his permission twice before she poured in the water. She then enjoyed pushing the wet sand, first using only one hand, but afterwards both where necessary. In the end she made a scene with mountains, rivers and lakes and therapist commented on the freedom inherent in such spacious country.

The therapist wondered if modelling with clay would give Miriam a better opportunity of expression, but in the event the use of clay did not carry them a great deal further, although it did bring to light Miriam's desire to know things. This suggested that if parents, relatives or teachers were able to talk to her, read to her or take her to places of interest and teach her history, folk-lore and things of cultural interest, her ability to acquire knowledge and so to read might be developed. At one difficult point the therapist had asked if she would like to go home, although the normal time for the interview was not up. Miriam replied, with little expression: 'It's all right.' The therapist remarked that she was unable even to answer this question and that she could not make any decisions, as if something inside her was saying that it was wrong to take any initiative.

One day Miriam said that she was likely to be going into a higher section of the class and this she both wanted and, to a slight extent, feared. She did, in fact, go into this higher section and we learned that her reading age was now approaching her mental age. She also became more animated in treatment sessions; she elected to paint and she spoke of her prowess in horse riding and of her ascendancy over a less successful friend.

The nominal objective of therapy, a substantial improvement in reading capacity, was being attained.

At the present stage of development of child guidance the chief interest of cases such as the above is their demonstration of reading disability as but one, although perhaps the most practically important, facet of emotional disturbance and the argument they provide for the provision of psychological treatment.

Mirror writing is best regarded as a minor degree of reading (or writing) disability. Hermann points to the considerable factor of anxiety which child sufferers from dyslexia sometimes experience. On a lighter note, we may look first for simple explanations before invoking more serious causes. An intelligent child was getting persistently bad results in arithmetic and neither he nor his teachers could discover the reason. His mother decided to study the matter with him. She discovered that if he was doing an addition sum and the total for one column came to, say, 56, instead of putting down 6 and carrying 5 to the next column, he put down 5 and carried 6. To point this out to him was all that was necessary.

As regards the treatment of reading disability one wants to be sure, to begin with, that there is no demonstrable neurological lesion. This excluded, the psychological and psychiatric investigations should be no less thorough than for any other disability and if stresses are discovered these should be dealt with. Unless the child's reading improves with this kind of attention at the clinic, there will be a case for remedial teaching at the hands of a qualified remedial teacher. The almost traditional tendency to relate stammer or dyslexia to left-handedness or to dominance of the left eye (right cerebral dominance) has not been therapeutically gainful.

Mental subnormality, backwardness and educational subnormality. The treatment of these conditions, as such, obviously is not a child guidance clinic responsibility, but the handling of related problems may become so. Children who are poorly endowed intellectually are not immune from the other ills that affect the psyche and problems of behaviour disorder or of anxiety may call for our help. Where play therapy within the clinic is undertaken we are apt to find that those children whose intelligence quotients are in the low 80's or less cannot make the same response to interpretive or explanatory techniques, but they can respond to therapy at the level of making a relationship which will give the child support and will make him happier and better able to adjust to the circumstances of his life. Nor is the value of the social worker's contribution with the child's mother to be underestimated. The clinic may also play a useful part in making recommendations for admission to a particular hospital unit or to an appropriate residential school or otherwise, and parents and colleagues who are responsible for the child's care are able to rely on us for help of this kind. The educational psychologist's contribution within the child's school will usually take the form of discussing with teachers their problems, and can be of much value.

In dealing with backwardness the importance of remedial teaching for those children whose work is below the level of their intellectual competence is now so well established that the education department which does not have such a service is in danger of being regarded as backward itself. Although this service is usually outside the domain of the child guidance clinic, the educational psychologist may contribute in various ways to its efficiency.

When a child who is not progressing well has been referred either to the clinic or to the educational psychologist when she has visited his school, we naturally regard it as our first objective not only to ascertain his I.Q. but also to decide whether and how far emotional difficulties are at the back of the problem.

The handling of educationally subnormal (usually spoken of as 'E.S.N.') children is largely a matter for the education department, and the E.S.N. special school, whether residential or day, is, in the writer's experience, usually staffed by people who work wonders with these children. Sometimes the help of the clinic is called for concerning E.S.N. children who are showing severe behaviour disturbance or are seriously delinquent, but such cases seem to be, if anything, less numerous proportionately than they are in the case of normally intelligent girls and boys. Another area where difficulties sometimes arise is in the case of E.S.N. children too young to go to the special school but who present special difficulties to the teacher in the infant or primary school. The position varies from area to area, but few E.S.N. schools take children under the age of seven and some not until they are several years older than this. There is no particular formula for dealing with this problem, both administrative and clinical in its nature, and which therefore provides a certain scope for the initiative of psychologist or psychiatrist.

We were asked to see a girl of fourteen (I.Q. 59) because of misbehaviour at school, mostly of a sexual kind, such as showing her genital area to boys in the cloakroom. It seemed that the school health department had tried to arrange for Olivia to go to an E.S.N. residential school, but that her parents had refused, and as there was no day E.S.N. school in the area she was attending the ordinary school. It might have been better had the school health department asked for the help of the child guidance clinic when the negotiations for the residential school were going on, but that is a matter of opinion. Olivia was an attractive child and was not unfriendly, though in the clinic she was inhibited. This inhibited behaviour was not characteristic of her attitudes at school and outside, where she was said to associate freely and irresponsibly with other children.

Olivia's mother was concerned for her daughter. We thought she was perhaps too encouraging of the child's dependence on her, but on the whole the relationships existing at home appeared to be satisfactory. She was clearly resentful that the problem could not have been more tactfully handled by the headmistress. We, for our part, wondered why the teaching staff of a school with which we already had a cordial understanding over another matter did not think to get in touch with us instead of letting things go the long route of an 'official' letter from the principal school medical officer.

After Olivia and her mother had left us we decided, at our clinic staff conference, that the best plan would be for the psychiatrist to go along to have a talk with the headmistress in the school. This he did; the discussion was friendly and enlightening and his next decision was to see the girl's mother and father together. To them he explained how the mother was allowing herself to worry about the situation and how unhelpful worrying could be. He also pointed out how mother and headmistress were working apart and perhaps not understanding each other and he suggested a combined meeting of parents, headmistress and himself. At that interview the pyschiatrist initiated the exchange of views by saying what he saw to be the misunderstandings and he mentioned what were the mother's suspicions. A friendly and reasonably open talk followed; the psychiatrist commented as he saw fit and the girl's problems were discussed in an atmosphere in which there could be a fairly free ventilation of opinion. Two and a half months afterwards we asked the headmistress about Olivia's progress. She said that Olivia had been quieter since even before the last interview and that she herself had heard of no further unsatisfactory incidents since that interview. Her concern now was as to what would happen after she left school in less than a year's time, and it could well be that we in the clinic should have to co-operate with the youth employment officer and with the parents once more in helping them to accept what might be unpleasant facts.

Clumsy children are a group whose awkwardness of movement gives the impression of impaired muscular co-ordination and whose want of grace in performance may be matched by a lack of lucidity in verbal expression, yet whose intelligence level is average. The disability may be regarded as a limitation of constitutional endowment which has been aggravated by emotional factors or we may regard some of the cases as likely to have been determined entirely by emotional difficulties. Work done on this condition was reviewed in a leading article[73] in 1962 and there was a subsequent contribution by Burns.[74] The conclusions so far reached by the various authors suggested that clumsiness in children was generally due to such organic factors as delayed maturation, anoxia at birth, parietal lobe lesions or minimal cerebral palsy, while Burns's cases were related to torsion spasm and were treatable with artane (benzhexol). This group of conditions is too disparate to allow us to regard clumsiness as a clinical entity, but their existence underlines the need for both psychological testing and neurological examination as well as psychiatric assessment.

We do, however, occasionally see in the clinic a child whose intelligence is in the average range or above, who does not appear to suffer from any neurological disability, but who is habitually clumsy or awkward in manner and behaviour.

Such a boy was Clement, who was referred to us at the age of nine and a half, his disability having been discovered at school during a survey undertaken by one of the remedial teachers. He was an only child, I.Q. 119, was clumsy in his movements, seemed to live in a dream world of his own, had difficulty in getting to sleep and occasionally had temper tantrums and a tic.

In treatment he displayed inhibition, he took no initiative, it was necessary to suggest that he might make a sand scene, might paint something or might play with toy animals. Even then going was slow, because, for example, he would not know what to paint and he had to be coaxed in order to give him courage to begin. A practical difficulty was that when I did get him to talk it was difficult for me to understand what he said and unless I spoke carefully and slowly he did not understand me. I decided to take him into the garden and found that he was much more agile outside than one would have expected.

In one interview he drew a sea and air battle. From this he was able to say a little about people he would like to throttle and he acted this with his hands. He said they would call each other names and then they might like to strangle him, but he could not mention any of the names, presumably as these were taboo.

Four and a half years after our first meeting Clement came back with his mother at our invitation. She said that he had progressed well and that she was satisfied with his developments, but despite some measure of improvement had had not yet gained an ascendancy over his environment.

Sonia was thirteen when she was referred to us on account of restless, jerky, clumsy behaviour. She had one older brother and with an I.Q. of 108 she had achieved a grammar-school place. Three years earlier she had had St Vitus's dance; she had seen the pediatrician both then and just about the time when she came to see us, and it appeared that on neither occasion had he considered that any serious physical disability was present. She had affectionate parents and a good home.

Sonia's present symptoms were these. She had difficulty in getting to sleep. She had moods when she felt unhappy and twice recently she had come home from school, crying, having fallen out with friends. She confided in the cat. Her arms and legs were 'very jumpy', she was wont to grimace, her walking was irregular and she had fallen two or three times at school. For a few weeks she was unable to use her right hand and I noticed that, as she painted in the clinic, she did so with her left hand and that her right arm hung by her side. Her headmistress said she had no idea what to do with a ball. Interestingly enough she had for years been able to ride a horse and could even jump when riding.

No physical lesion was discovered to account for these things, but there was some evidence of emotional stress, so that the inferential diagnosis was that of emotionally produced clumsiness of movement. Because Sonia considered that there was very little wrong except for her difficulty in getting to sleep, I thought that treatment might not be easy. Yet it was not too difficult to discuss her problems with her and at the end of three months the difficulties had largely disappeared. Six years later I had a letter from Sonia telling me how busy and interested she was and how much she was enjoying life.

The problems of gifted children. It may come as a surprise that highly gifted children not only may have special problems but that they are also peculiarly vulnerable to being misunderstood. It has long been popularly suspected that genius has a rather high statistical correlation with nervous breakdown, and it is probable that highly intelligent children are prone to be more delicate in their emotional poise – less 'tough' in their social contacts we may say – than is the average child. It is, however, the second aspect of their problem, the risk they run of being misjudged, which usually is the more important.

It is a fact that within the community generally the more intelligent people tend to marry others who are also of high intellect, while it is a circumstance of heredity that bright parents are, on the average, likely to have bright children. Gifted children have, therefore, a good statistical chance of being born into families that are intellectually well endowed. This, however, is not always so, and even where it is, the gifted child may be so far above the expected level even in a *milieu* of quite intelligent relatives, that his capabilities are missed. If the child's special abilities have not been recognized at home, at school the risk will be even greater and the gifted child may become a 'problem' child. Branch and Cash have provided an arresting study of this subject.[75]

The gifted child whose parents are unimaginative may find that the spirit of his eager enquiries is stifled by the indifference of those around him to capacities of which they are unaware. If, on the other hand, he has received encouragement at home he will, by the time he goes to school, already be able to read and will wish to learn about things that are quite beyond the grasp of the other children in the class and beyond the expectation of the teacher. The risk now is that he will become frankly bored, will lose all interest in applying himself to the simplicities of subject-matter that he mastered long ago and that his performance will fall away to almost nothing. Uncomprehending pedagogues may dub him as slothful, dull or both, and his behaviour may deteriorate, bringing down upon him further contumely, until he is reduced to a state of bewilderment in the face of a situation in which he can find no meaning.

It may be hoped that the picture will seldom be so black or the potential consequences so ruinous, but this risk to a gifted child is there and the existence of such a state of affairs is always a possibility when it is reported that a child is, unaccountably, doing badly in class. The child's safeguards are the vigilance of teachers, the ready awareness of the educational psychologist and his colleagues in the clinic, the co-operation of parents and the purposeful intention of the education service as a whole to make necessary provision for those children who are gifted so that they may become leaders. A gifted child who has fallen behind may require from the clinic a period of treatment with a view to the restoration of his shaken self-confidence.

CHAPTER VIII
Behaviour Disorders and Delinquency

Behaviour disorder is a useful term with which to comprise a wide variety of behaviour difficulties, ranging from symptoms that are obviously the result of anxiety at one end of the scale to what is frankly delinquent at the other. Ultimately nearly all behaviour will be found to be the result of anxieties which are repressed. Aggressive behaviour which is marked by violence, destructiveness or an excessive degree of mischief will raise a question as to the possible presence of brain damage or of epilepsy. In some behaviour disorders the E.E.G. shows an excess of slow activity, but the meaning of this is uncertain. Equally important is the psychologist's assessment of intelligence and of attitudes, but it will turn out in the end that the great majority have arisen through stresses within the family relationship. It is towards better understanding in this area that treatment will mainly be directed.

A disturbing form of aggressive behaviour which one meets occasionally is *destruction of clothes*, usually by cutting with scissors or a knife. More often than not it is his own clothes that the child attacks in this way, but one little boy used to come downstairs very early in the morning and cut slits in his father's coat. In my experience children who behave in this way are suffering from strong feelings of rejection and the chief aim of therapy will be to discover where the fault lies and to improve relations within the family.

Joseph, the boy who cut his father's coat, was seven and a half years old when he came to us, but almost two years earlier he had been to another child guidance clinic. The complaint was of behaviour disorder – stealing and lying, waking up during the night and raiding the larder, stealing sweets, cutting father's coat, lighting fires in the house and burning clothes, destroying toys of siblings, attacking bigger boys and fighting at home. A sizeable indictment! He was now also in the way of getting the blame for things that he had not done. His I.Q. we assessed at 91 (a test at the previous clinic had made it 86). He was the fourth of six children.

Joseph was not a wanted baby. His mother had thyroid trouble when pregnant; she did not want another child at that time and in his early years she was irritable and impatient. She was at times depressed, especially during her pregnancies. His father was a regular soldier and the family were abroad till Joseph was three. He was a moody individual who had found readjustment in civilian life difficult after returning to the United Kingdom. Money was short and the family's total load of anxiety was appreciable, but so far as we could discover there seemed to have been little trouble with any of the other children.

Joseph's mother said he always seemed to be the odd one out. There were battles over toilet training; he soiled till he was nearly three years old and he played with faeces. In a more permissive family setting it would have been a healthy sign if his mother could have accepted this without anxiety and the child could do it without guilt. In actual fact she was punitive for a time, after which she ignored it until Joseph asked for a long tie. Promised this as a reward, he became and remained clean. He used to take things from shops and this had continued at school. He had food fads – as do many children. Since he had been a toddler he used to wander about the house in the early morning, emptied things into the lavatory pan and 'created havoc' in the pantry and in his father's desk. Joseph said he preferred his father to his mother, but he showed envy of his father's status and he became distressed if his mother were ill. At school he was a fairly good mixer, but he tended to be aggressive and to fall out easily. His work and concentration were poor. Therapy within the clinic for Joseph resolved itself largely into a relationship-making series of interviews, and this, coupled with, what was still more important, a vigorous effort on the social worker's part in interviews with the mother to achieve more caring parental attitudes, produced a level of better-adjusted behaviour, although the position remained precarious. Shortly after this the family moved from our area and we were unable to trace them later on.

Where *adolescent* behaviour disorder is concerned moditen (fluphenazine hydrochlor.) is reputedly a useful sedative, but one on which patients may become dependent. Several workers have found that haloperidol is valuable as an adjunct to other forms of therapy when dealing with severe behaviour disorder. Dosage: Haloperidol – 0·5 mg. in two divided doses in the first day and gradually increased over a period of eight days to 3·0 mg. a day, and continued on this dosage. Benzhexol hydrochloride, 2·0 mg. daily in two divided doses, is given along with the haloperidol in order to avoid side effects. There appears to be no serious contra-indication to the use of this drug for a few weeks on end. Possible adverse effects of administration over a long period should be borne in mind.[76]

Temper tantrums are so common that, unless they are severe or frequent or persist into later childhood, there is no cause for undue concern. As a first-aid method of treatment parents are encouraged to accept them as something which the child cannot control and to avoid themselves becoming either anxious or angry. This does not mean that mother is indifferent, for she stands by her child, and she may at times decide to be firm in refusing to allow, for example, attacks on herself or damage to things of value. The child will gain from this support. Sometimes a child, during a phase of temper, destructiveness or persistent girning complaint may inwardly feel so guilty that he desires punishment, and in such a case the reasoned smack may have its place. The author's preference is for control through the moral relationship a parent has with his or her child, rather than for punishment, and if there are any punishments they are within the framework of that relationship. It is only if such measures fail, or the parents are incapable of such understanding behaviour, that treatment within the clinic will come into the picture.

Just as an excess of restrictiveness on the part of parents may produce emotional stress within the child, so unbridled freedom will cause anxiety. The child is afraid of his own aggressions and of the damage, fantasied or real, which he may do, and he needs to have behind him a loving but controlling parent. If parents can, without being angry or anxious themselves, set a limit to the child's outbursts, they will be fostering his development of self-confidence. In one of our industrial areas our health visitors have noticed in recent years that that mothers of immigrant, mainly Jamaican, babies train them to sit inactive in their cots indefinitely. The visitors' impression is that this does not seem to be harmful and that the reason perhaps is that mother is constantly present.

Wandering away from home is a relatively common symptom, and while the odd occasion is probably of no great importance, persistent wandering or running off betokens a serious breakdown in relationships which calls urgently for treatment. In a number of such cases there has been a real measure of neglect on parents' part to consider their child's interests, and this is one of the kinds of cases which may best be dealt with by arranging for the child to go to a residential school for maladjusted children.

Delinquency. It is useful in practice to regard as delinquent those children who have committed acts which the law regards as being offences or crimes, but with the exception of truancy. Pearce[77] quotes Burt as saying that a child is to be regarded as a delinquent when his

BEHAVIOUR DISORDER

anti-social tendencies appear so grave that he becomes, or ought to become, the subject of official action. In modern terms official action may mean referral to a child guidance clinic or substitute agency such as the probation service. We should not regard telling lies as a part of the delinquency. If a child steals it would be almost naïve to expect that he would be able to tell the truth about it. These children have strong feelings of guilt and if they cannot avoid committing misdemeanours they will seldom be able to confess them.

The misdemeanours which we mostly come across are *stealing, behaviour disorders, wilful damage, arson*, and among older boys *sexual offences* and the *taking away and driving of motor cars*. Prostitution and the loose habits which come close to it are a serious form of delinquency among older girls, even when they do not actually contravene the law. The driving of motor cars and motor cycles without permission by persons who have not the necessary skill is a dangerous type of offence which has become uncomfortably common. Pearce says: 'The most common form of sexual delinquency is corrupting by talk', and: 'The more serious forms are those in which children live in prostitution and occasionally they are boys.'

As regards causes, the formerly held idea that criminals were a special physical type has been shown to be without foundation, and even where a known physical factor such as epilepsy operates there are frequently emotional reasons also to account for the disordered behaviour. Intelligence is not an important factor causatively, although it has a bearing on treatment. The recent discovery that an undue proportion of criminal men have an extra Y chromosome is disturbing and gives cause for some alteration in our thinking.[78]

What stood out most in my own study was that delinquent children are nervous children, that is to say that apart from the delinquent behaviour there were other features for which the child might reasonably have been brought to the child guidance clinic.[79] Michaels found a relationship between delinquency and bed-wetting and Knox discovered that many members of the prison population at Camp Hill Prison gave histories of screaming fits, severe nightmares or bed-wetting.[80] Home conditions are of significance and from the above study it appeared that the majority of delinquent children come from homes that are not happy, are in other ways unsatisfactory, or where the child-parent relationships leave a good deal to be desired.

The present century has seen a great increase in affluence in most European or Western countries and following in the train of this affluence there have been increases in criminality and notably in delinquent behaviour among adolescents. The demand for higher material standards has tended to oust the *emotional* care of children from the pride of place which it used to have in the mental economy of the average mother. There is a tendency to compensate by material gifts for the parents' inability to give of themselves and to substitute material advantages within the home to offset the disadvantages of having both parents out at work. A materialistic attitude of mind displaces the self-giving love which is the true source of a child's happiness in a disturbingly high proportion of homes. Poverty is not a major cause of delinquency and hard circumstances can have the opposite effect if they bind the members of a family to each other.

Stealing is generally the most obtrusive of the manifestations of delinquency. It is useful to divide cases of stealing into three groups. In the first are those children whose stealing is done at home and by themselves when alone. In the second group are those who steal outside their homes, but who do so alone. The third group comprises those children who steal outside their homes in company with other children. There must, of course, be a certain amount of overlapping, but generally speaking those in the first group are those children who have the greatest amount of feeling of insecurity and of rejection, while their aggression is certainly less to the fore even if it resides, as indeed it must, in their unconscious. The third group tend to be the most aggressive, although deeper feelings of rejection underlie their aggressive emotions. The middle group tend to lie somewhere between the other two on this rejection-aggression scale. All have feelings of guilt, a point which is far too little recognized by most adult authorities.

The motivation for the stealing is usually a feeling of rejection. A good deal of this is usually conscious, but one must recognize that there is also a deep well of unconscious emotion. It is found in practice that this feeling of being rejected corresponds fairly closely with the emotional realities of the situation and that the parents of these children have, wittingly or otherwise, denied them much of the love they needed, whether this has arisen from psychological maladjustment on the parents' part, a materialistic attitude in the home, a tendency to favour a sibling or some other form of want of parental care. This is not always the case and stealing can arise from sibling jealousy or some other distortion at an unconscious level of the child's own assessment of the real emotional situation within his home, but if we look far enough we shall usually find that a want of consideration of the little child as an individual who has a right to unselfish love and whose needful desires should take precedence over the comfort of his parents has damaged his relationship with them. Even though stealing sometimes will arise from internal factors such as an apparently endogenous depression, or external ones in the form of social pressure by companions, these are exceptions.

From the feeling of rejection will have stemmed a wild and enhanced desire to obtain love, and if this eventuates in stealing, then the symptom will be by way of compensation. Thefts from mother's purse and stealing of food are the more obvious examples, but this motivation operates throughout stealing generally. Equally the child who feels rejected will be resentful and perhaps it is this, more than anything else, which provides the drive, unconscious in its nature as it is persistent in its purpose, that perpetuates the stealing. Stealing is thus an aggressive act.

Such factors have to be recognized as a background to any programme of treatment. The therapist will understand that the child usually cannot help stealing any more than he can keep himself from skipping and jumping, or any more, we might say, than some adults can keep themselves from smoking. Our task is to enable the child to alter his feelings, to make him happier, so that our treatment is not specifically aimed at the stealing. The child's need to find good relationships is the superlative consideration. If these good relationships can be effected at home with his parents, this will be quite the best result. Sometimes, where this is not possible something worth while and lasting may be gained through a good and continuing relationship with the therapist in the clinic, or with the probation officer. This can then extend to an improved situation with teachers and others at school and even in the child's, in this case, unsatisfactory home. Where this has failed to materialize there usually remains a reasonable chance that the environment provided by a residential school for maladjusted children – an approved school sometimes – will allow this essential relationship to be formed with members of the staff as parental figures. One can never afford to lose sight of the fact that, with it all, however blatant the stealing may sometimes appear to be, it is always accompanied by a substantial amount of guilt feeling and the extent to which this is conscious varies from one child to another. It is the oppressive force of this guilt which makes it often so difficult for the child to discuss or even to admit the misbehaviour.

Margaret, aged seventeen, was a girl of average intelligence who had indulged in solitary stealing, both at home and outside, during a period of four years. She was the eldest of five children and the family appeared, by and large, to be a happy middle-class household. There was some evidence that her father, who seemed to be an easy-going individual in a family dominated by the mother, had transferred too much of his affection to Margaret's younger sisters. Margaret had left school at the age of fourteen and a half and was working as a clerk. She was smartly dressed and looked older than she was, but showed marked inhibition of emotional expression. She was not easy to talk to. She evidently craved for love, but she withdrew from making love relationships. Although the origins of the problem were not fully clear, there were grounds for suspecting that a faulty relationship with her mother had developed early in her life and that, unconsciously, she felt rejected by her father.

The girl was seen in twelve interviews and it was at first difficult to have any communion with her. A drawing which she did of a dancing couple allowed the therapist to make some entry into discussing the feeling part of her life. Once he got to know her a little she was able to place a small measure of trust in his intentions and from that beginning it was possible to move on to an exploration of the kind of feeling situation which existed at home. An improved relationship with her parents resulted and her delinquency receded. Three years afterwards we heard from her doctor that she had been married for a year and that there had been no further trouble.

Where *sexual offences* are concerned my own study of some forty boys whom I had treated on account of such misconduct has engendered a degree of optimism with regard to the probable outcome if their cases are handled imaginatively.[81] Doshay, in his much larger study, found that juvenile sexual offenders did not usually commit violations of the sexual code in later life. A sub-group within his series, who had as children committed other offences as well as the sexual ones, did slightly less well as regards their later sexual behaviour.[82]

Indecent exposure, minor sexual assaults of the looking (voyeurism) and touching (indecent assault) type, attempts at intercourse or partial intercourse with little girls and homosexual assaults by older boys upon younger boys – these all occur from time to time. An element of aggression may occasionally accompany this behaviour, but in boys of school age feelings of love are the prominent attitude and the behaviour is that of immature and insecure boys who are attempting to find for themselves sensual satisfaction. One must have regard to the love desires as the primary emotion even if selfish desire appears to be the only characteristic of their expression – e.g. in assaults on young children.

Boys who indulge in indecent exposure we may regard as typical of the group. They usually are timid, inhibited and shy. In treating them, and others in this group, it is worth remembering that their behaviour is a substitute for normal behaviour on the part of a boy who lacks the ability to achieve what he needs in an entirely healthy manner. I am inclined to discuss more general matters first and where the exposure is concerned I shall say that there must be a lot of boys who do it at one time or another and that I do not regard it as a particularly heinous offence. It is vital to conduct the therapy in a way which will enable the boy to believe that the therapist believes in him: in this manner he is helped to feel that he is as good as other people. Avoidance of anything that appears to be prying, coupled with the aim of bringing to the surface feelings about himself – a strong sense of guilt and unworthiness underlies the sexual behaviour and not a few are victims of unsatisfactory relationships at home – and about himself in relation to others will go some way towards providing an emotional atmosphere in which the growth of self-confidence is possible.

Denis, the older of two children in a professional family, was referred at the age of almost fourteen because he had been stealing ladies' underclothes. He also suffered from dyslexia. He would not accept the interpretation that he did this in order to make of himself a girl substitute and he even said that he did not want a girl, but this has to be seen as a defence by denial because he felt too guilty to admit his real sexual desires. Most of the second session was taken up by the painting of a winged horse and in a shy attempt to make a relationship Denis referred to the rain outside the window and said that his uncle was working in a garage that was visible in the distance. In the next interview we discussed the painting. The therapist said that the horse, flying alone, and being shy, was perhaps finding it difficult to get on with other horses, wishing to get away and yet having nowhere really to go. He wondered if Denis was lonely and if people did not understand him. Denis countered this by saying that when you caught a big fish – fishing was one of his hobbies – you had to act alone. The inner meaning of this must be that being involved with his sexual powers – very satisfying powers but difficult to control just like the big fish – he felt he must handle them unaided. The therapist afterwards asked if he had had any dreams, but none were forthcoming. The picture of the horse contained an object very like a nipple, and the therapist returned to the subject of the horse, saying that it seemed to be looking for something; there was no comfort in the clouds among which it was flying and maybe it was looking for a girl horse. As Denis had nothing to say, the therapist suggested a further painting and this time the subject of the picture Denis produced was a fire engine. The therapist said that the presence of a fire engine was indicative of something wrong and that in Denis's life this was likely to have something to do with girls. Denis tried to say that there was nothing wrong with him, but the therapist countered by asking why he was coming to see him, a doctor, if there were nothing wrong. Denis then admitted there was a problem and he agreed with the therapist's comment that he did not quite understand what, although it did relate to girls. The therapist said a little about girls, how they, too, were shy and had anxieties. He spoke of feelings in ourselves, how one half of a person felt good and the other half felt bad, of feelings that some of our impulses were silly or were naughty, and of the angry emotions – we feel afraid to let others know of these feelings and yet the truth is that others feel the same. Denis said virtually nothing, but seemed to grasp the therapist's meaning.

Several interviews had passed in this way when Denis told the therapist that he could now read well enough to do so for pleasure. The therapist talked about relationship difficulties, particularly about how it must seem to Denis that his mother and father did not always understand him or his needs. In the next interview the therapist spoke of difficulties in making relationships with girls, of his feelings of inferiority, of how other boys also had secret habits, and of masturbation, which he regarded as being sometimes a necessity in our social circumstances and as having a personal value as an outlet for emotion. A little later the therapist raised the issue of taking women's underclothes and Denis accepted dressing up and getting an erection, although he said he did not think that he masturbated. The therapist was content that his grasp of the meaning of his own situation in relation to other people was now such that he should be able to handle the force of his own emotions. A recent school report indicated considerable progress. To keep in touch for a while longer through widely spaced interviews seemed all that would now be necessary, and when Denis came to the clinic a year and nine months after his first attendance it was decided that no further contact was called for. The period of active treatment had begun six weeks after the initial attendance and had lasted for three months.

Transvestism, as the behaviour of men or youths who wear women's clothes is called, and the often associated practice of stealing women's underclothes or of collecting and hiding them, have come to our notice in the clinic so often that such behaviour on the part of boys, at least occasionally, must be fairly common. When it comes to treatment I usually say that I know that a good many boys do it at some time or another, thus allaying any fears the boy may have of being regarded as a pariah. I mostly try to enable the boy to see that what he actually is doing is to make a substitute girl for himself, because, either on account of his shyness or because girls are so difficult to get to know intimately, he cannot get a real one. Beyond this, little further mention or none may be made of the behaviour specifically, and the treatment aims rather to inculcate a greater feeling of self-confidence than to concentrate on activities which are symptomatic. Once a relationship has grown up between the boy and the therapist, the boy may ask him such questions as how to get a girl friend, and it may then be useful for the therapist to say something about the feelings and resultant attitudes of girls as well as helping the boy better to understand the origins of his own inadequacy. His relationship with the therapist, in inculcating in the boy a sense that someone believes in him, may be among the more important aspects of the treatment.

Affectionless children. Following the well-known work of Bowlby and others on maternal deprivation, we have used this term to describe those children who have been so deprived emotionally that they have lost the capacity to form affectionate relationships. These are the children from whom one expects the ranks of the adult psychopaths to be recruited and some, perhaps all, will show delinquent tendencies. Typical is the foster-child whose foster-mother is at first concerned to find that the baby can make no response to her affectionate caresses and is later distressed to discover that the growing child is purposelessly untruthful and is developing a tendency to perform meaningless acts of nastiness, such as one little girl who killed a kitten and denied all knowledge of it, but secreted the body in the drawer with her underclothes. An inability to conform to constructive discipline or to accept affectionate advances within the family is paralleled by a series of anti-social acts and unbecoming attitudes in a variety of situations.

Where treatment is concerned we have to face the fact that these children are so damaged that they cannot acquire the capacity to be loving, yet it would be intolerably negative to assume that we can do nothing for them. We are justified in hoping that therapy will enable some of them to become adjusted at least to the extent of acceptable living within the community, but unless a good therapeutic relationship can be made in the clinic it will have to be supplemented by residential school or even approved school later on.

Examination and report to the magistrates. Not least in importance among the services which the children's psychiatrist performs is that of making reports to the Court. At one of the writer's clinics it is the educational psychologist who sends the reports to the Court, but usually it is the psychiatrist who does so. We may ask why it is from us that this vital information is sought. In placing this responsibility upon the expert in child guidance society is showing an awareness that he is qualified by the depth of his understanding to make a

TREATMENT FOR CHILDREN

unique contribution. We are not the only people who care for children, but in the assessment of a child's need by a psychiatrist his complex-free personality, his training, skill and experience, the support which the clinic makes available to him and the time at his disposal, are all relevant.

If, after assessing the child and his environment, we favour an arrangement whereby he remains at home, we may usefully, but briefly, indicate what we see as the guide lines of therapy. If we have reason to believe, either from our previous handling if we already know the child, or on account of the conditions in his home, or because of adverse features of character that are already established in himself, that a particular boy or girl will not be able to make a good response to out-patient therapy or to probation, it will then usually be necessary to recommend some form of residential care.

The magistrates, in those cases where a report has been requested for the Court, will usually welcome a short statement in plain English and free from unnecessary detail of the factors operating at home, the circumstances of the child's wider environment and the features in himself which underlie the recommendations the psychiatrist is going to make for their consideration. Seldom indeed will it be a case of saying whether or not the child is responsible for his actions, the criminal responsibility so dear to adult forensic practice, but rather of indicating how his delinquent propensities are likely to be transformed into more socially acceptable patterns of behaviour. The Court will wish to know how good or how poor will be the prospects of the less disturbing forms of Court decision, such as conditional or absolute discharge, probation, child guidance, attendance centre order or a small fine, without, of course, specifically mentioning these alternatives unless to recommend one of them. Where such permissive measures are considered unlikely to prosper the psychiatrist should say briefly why and should indicate what he considers is likely to be best, approved school [83] for example, and he may usefully add what sort of conditions of control or understanding he believes to be necessary for this particular boy or girl. He is giving to the justices opinions based on his experience and training and on the special knowledge which the clinic has acquired. He should not presume to dictate, and any form of arrogance or of unconstructive criticism of the comments of others is quite out of place, but the magistrates, for their part, would be doing less than justice to the child if they did not pay careful attention to what he had said. It is regrettable if the Court has to receive conflicting reports from psychiatrist, probation officer, remand home superintendent or other professional adviser. Sometimes

BEHAVIOUR DISORDER

the psychiatrist is put in a position where he cannot avoid this happening, but it is vastly better if some sort of conference can take place beforehand so that any major differences of viewpoint are ironed out before recommendations are written down and placed in the hands of the clerk to the justices.

CHAPTER IX

Problems Involving Sexual Development, the Integrity of the Family and Social Integration

Masturbation to excess is probably one of the less frequent forms of disturbed behaviour. We are not here considering masturbation to a degree that is common enough with average children and with which parents may deal by ignoring it or, if it seems to call for attention, by looking at themselves to see if there are ways in which they are falling short of meeting their child's emotional needs. We are thinking of those cases where the schoolmistress is bothered because a child masturbates continuously and more or less openly. It has been my experience that those children are always suffering from some form of emotional loss and that the shortcoming lies in the degree of selfless love that their parents are able to give to them.

Parents can be plausible in this, as in other conditions, and the mother of a five-year-old boy who was attending a private school and whose mistress complained of this problem, was herself cool and unforthcoming as regards there being any difficulties in the domestic situation. It was far from easy to find the underlying fault until the family doctor explained that the family were a hierarchial group, severely dominated by grandfather, and that they were the kind of people who would pay their bills only short of going to prison in default. So far as treatment was concerned, little more could be done than try to get it across to mother that in some way this child felt that he was being kept short of love and that life was for him, in the event, rather joyless. Enquiries which our social worker made almost one year, and eight years, afterwards, gave the impression that the boy was making satisfactory progress, but a year after the second of these enquiries he hanged himself from a tree.

Homosexual behaviour need be a cause for concern only if it is persistent or if it appears to be becoming a way of life for someone already approaching, or in, his middle teens. Treatment, in the case of younger boys, will comprise an attempt at sympathetic and tactful

SOCIO-SEXUAL DIFFICULTIES

adjustment of their circumstances and, one hopes, an avoidance of the attitude of mind which implies that grown-ups know what is best. Psychotherapy for a teenager will obviously be dependent upon the patient's co-operation.

Transsexuality is a condition in which the patient wishes intensely to become a member of the opposite sex and to be accepted as such and these patients may believe that nature has somehow transposed things so that they have the wrong anatomical parts for their actual sex. They are thus different from the homosexual, who does not usually have any desire for his sex to be altered. It is said that some abnormality of behaviour is usually apparent by the age of ten and that a growing conviction of anomaly exists in the early teens. Most are boys. Treatment presents a tricky problem. Psychotherapy, founded upon a purposefully sincere attempt to enter into the young person's feelings and thus to be able to share with him a true understanding of his difficulties, will enable the therapist to go along with him in a relationship that is meaningful.[84]

Crushes are a normal part of development for some girls and their desirability is to be called in question only if there is excessive preoccupation with the lady who is the object of the crush. Lewis has said of adolescent love affairs that what they are is the child's projection of all that he or she would most like to become, upon the loved one.[85] Efforts at psychotherapy should avoid the temptation to be interfering or to pry beyond what the girl is willing to reveal. *Festina lente* is a good maxim for therapy in teenage matters of this kind.

Pregnancy in an unmarried girl. Occasionally the children's psychiatrist has to face up to the question as to whether he would be justified in recommending a therapeutic termination of pregnancy in a girl who has been referred to him. The more permissive attitude of recent legislation will hardly alter the necessity to adhere to sound psychological principles, an adherence which was quite possible under the old law following Bourne's famous stand thirty years ago. A girl just under the age of sixteen became pregnant and her doctor referred her to me with the idea that I might be able to recommend termination. A year earlier her mother had been my patient; she had not continued her treatment for as long as I wished, but I knew of the considerable domestic stress under which the girl had grown up and which was still a characteristic of her present environment. She was emotionally insecure, her adjustment, domestically and socially, was unsatisfactory, so that there was a reasonable case for recommending psychiatric treatment. It was my opinion that the girl's poor emotional stability would be further undermined by having a baby and that this would also militate against the chances of her being materially helped by treatment. Under these circumstances termination of the pregnancy was recommended and was carried out. The police were interested in this case, because the mother of another girl had complained to them about the boy's behaviour towards her daughter, and in this way they came to know of our girl, who had been under the age of consent. After investigation they did not institute proceedings regarding the termination of the pregnancy.

Although a journey of twenty miles each way was involved each time, the girl subsequently attended my clinic for a couple of years, at frequencies which I considered satisfactory. She became the first of my child patients ever to send me a box of her own wedding cake, a year or two afterwards, and still later my wife and I had the pleasure of visiting her and her husband in their new home in South Africa.

Many of these girls who become pregnant have not been seeking a mature sexual relationship but have simply been in need of someone to love them. If the pregnancy has been terminated, subsequent treatment will start from the therapist's realization of this.

Unless there have been special circumstances, of which rape is the obvious example, to warrant termination of pregnancy in an adolescent, any decision to recommend it must be made against a background of knowledge of such factors as these. An emotionally deprived girl may have been, unconsciously, attempting to prove to herself her femininity; she may have been rebelling against a state of parental hegemony from which her psyche could find no other way of escape; she may already value the embryo in her womb as an extension of herself the destruction of which she would (unconsciously now, perhaps, but more purposefully after the surgical act had been performed) regard as infanticide, and she may be ill motivated to cooperate in any subsequent therapy. Hidden resentments and a sense that she has been violated may be additional and cogent reasons for a repetition of the pregnancy. Termination can seldom be justified unless it can be integrated as a part of therapy. Social considerations may be of some importance and the probable well-being or otherwise of the unborn child is to be weighed in the balance, but now that legislation which has been enacted permits surgical abortion on social grounds those in psychiatric care of children will have to be wary that they are not led up the garden path into a plot of psychic thistles and nettles.

The problem of *venereal disease* is not irrelevant to adolescent psychiatry especially because the evidence suggests that there has been a slight recent increase in its incidence among young people. Catterall has pointed out that anti-social behaviour in teenage girls is usually sexually orientated, and he stresses the importance of teenagers being made fully aware of the hazards of pre-marital sexual intercourse and being protected from them in as many ways as possible.[86] To have the right psychological attitude towards loving is probably the most valuable form of protection.

Loss of parents and the integrity of the family. The children's psychiatrist may be asked to help in connection with certain factual circumstances which vitally affect the child's happiness and welfare and which are, therefore, quite properly the concern of the child guidance service. These are misfortunes which inevitably involve separation from one or both parents and the issues are so wide that we can deal here only with salient features. We shall consider *loss of parents, step-parents, foster-parents,* children permanently in *residential homes, adoption, custody* and *access* by the displaced parent.

Where loss of one or both parents through death, desertion, divorce or otherwise is concerned we must expect the child to go through a period of mourning, which may be prolonged, and this is to be accepted and the child allowed to be alone with that part of his grief which he does not wish to share. Sometimes the grief, too painful to contemplate, is repressed, and we have a superficially bright child whose emotional responses lack depth and whose personality has become a mere shell of its former rich substance, and minor behaviour disturbances may become frequent. If treatment in the clinic is undertaken it will need to be cautious, based on making a relationship with the child. References to the parent who has died or has gone are made tangentially as they arise in play or paintings, but direct comment had better await the child's own statement.

Usually the remaining parent or whoever is caring for the child will be the appropriate therapist and the rôle of the child psychiatrist that of counsellor. A relative, such as aunt, uncle or grandparent, who is of the same sex as the parent the child has lost, may be encouraged to play a part in his life. It is good for the child if his lost parent can be talked about sometimes in the home, naturally, as anyone else is spoken about. The loss can be exceedingly hard for the child to bear and it is a help to him if we can give him a religious faith in the idea that Mummy or Daddy is living in Heaven and may even be able to see us. A belief in this immortality has supported mankind through the ages, and even if many adults today are genuinely unable to accept it, it would be a mistake to deny it to our children, especially at such a time of stress.

Step-parents are beset by unavoidable pitfalls however much they may love their stepchildren. It is equally true that the coming of an affectionate step-parent to the deprived family will benefit the

TREATMENT FOR CHILDREN

children greatly, but his or her expression of love may be met by surprising resistance even from children who have everything to gain from it on a conscious level; it is the unconscious resentments that can be the barrier to harmony.[87]

A boy whose father has died may well have become inordinately possessive of his mother and he may resent deeply and unreasoningly a stepfather who appears as a rival for his mother's affections. One such boy refused to call his stepfather by any name indicating fatherhood. From postwar experience we learned much of the strong hostilities felt by young children against the return of their father, whom they barely remembered if at all and who to them was an interloper who usurped their position with mother. No less strong antagonisms will be felt by stepchildren. An intelligent girl became excessively possessive of her father after her mother's death and when, at the age of sixteen, she found that he was contemplating marriage, she could meet this challenge only with total, blind opposition.

Loyalty to the dead parent may make the step-parent unacceptable and what makes this aspect of things particularly ineluctable is the circumstance that the child remembers the dead parent not as he was in real life but instead has the vision of an idealized parent, so that the unfortunate stepmother or stepfather is judged against the standard of this super-human image. Recently we had in treatment a little girl who gave to her stepfather every credit for his considerateness to her. Yet she was in a state of bewilderment and depression following her father's death in a road accident in which all the family had been involved many months earlier, so that her response was unspontaneous and at best an acceptance at conscious level. To form a good relationship with a child who is thus nervously ill will require a greater capacity for empathy than most people possess. Where divorce, rather then death, is the background the issues are unlikely to be less complicated.

Therapy within the clinic for such a child, assuming it has been decided that this is the proper course to adopt, will require an appreciation of the irreplaceable nature of what has been lost and a realization that time, rather than treatment, will be the ultimate healer. It is helpful to talk, and to encourage her to talk, of her father as he was, especially as this is something that is likely to be too little encouraged at home. But one would not press her to talk if she does not wish to. The child may reject the therapist, ignore him, read a book or remain speechless, and it is then important that she should see that the therapist accepts this behaviour as being natural under the circumstances. The therapist will have a patient understanding of her need to mourn – her family may have found this hard to tolerate

SOCIO-SEXUAL DIFFICULTIES

at home – and the clinic atmosphere will be accepting of such an attitude. The therapist should be under no pressure of anxiety to alter the child's attitudes or her behaviour in this respect.

In difficulties such as these and also in dealing with problems arising from placement with *foster-parents* it will usually be the psychiatrist's most profitable contribution to counsel the parents rather than to take the children for treatment, though there will be exceptions and sometimes a treatment relationship with the therapist will make all the difference in enabling the domestic situation to become stabilized. Where problems arise in *residential homes* counselling is of special value, a matter which we shall consider later when discussing the relationship between residential schools and the child guidance clinic.[88]

A child who is going to be *adopted* is likely to have less loving care from his mother in the earliest days and weeks of his life than a baby who is born under happier circumstances. On the other hand, adopting parents have usually been 'vetted' by someone in order to ensure that their emotional and cultural standards are of at least average merit. They are unlikely to do less than their level best for the little one whom they have taken into their family. In the clinic we have seen adopted children who have developed severe behaviour disorder or delinquency without what seemed to be sufficient reason to account for it, often enough to raise the question as to whether irreparable emotional damage may not have been done in the early weeks, before the child was taken over.[89] If this is true it will suggest that when adopted children with problems are brought to the clinic we should regard these problems with special concern. This may involve a greater urgency in treatment, a more cautious prognosis, and in some cases, paradoxical though it may appear, a greater readiness to employ residential measures for those who are seriously maladjusted.

Sometimes the child psychiatrist is approached regarding matters of *legal custody* and *access* by the parent who does not have the child's custody. A variety of problems can arise under this head and the Court is empowered to take decisions that are of great importance to the child's happiness and his future. The following are examples of legal issues in which the psychiatrist is expected to play a part.

The father of a little girl was discovered to have indulged in sex play with her and with one or two other young girls, to the extent, so far as we were aware, of touching their private parts. He was, in fact, put on probation for these offences, but his daughter was taken from home and sent to a children's home, where she remained for years. No psychiatrist was asked to give an opinion to the Court and no appeal was made. There were reasons for doubting the wisdom of both the above legal decisions, especially the latter, and the psychiatrist might, given the opportunity, have adduced strong grounds for interfering less drastically with the child's liberty.

The second type of case arises from the circumstance that the Courts have power nowadays to allow a child to be adopted even without the mother's consent or to be or remain in the custody of persons other than his parents and contrary to their wishes. The Court will tend to favour, other things being equal, the established tradition that the parents' rights in these matters are paramount. The psychiatrist should have sympathy for this natural tendency, but if he is convinced that another arrangement is in the child's interests he is right to state his opinion clearly. We are entitled to be listened to as experts, and if we avoid taking any unfair advantage of this, but say just what we believe genuinely, the Courts are nearly always prepared to give us a fair hearing.[90]

A further kind of difficulty occasionally arises where parents are divorced or separated and where the mother has custody of the children and the father right of access. These arrangements seem usually to work smoothly enough, but if the father is unsympathetic or is mentally unstable, afternoons spent with him may be a considerable burden to a child, and if they involve the loss of a Saturday afternoon's play every fortnight, so much the worse. The machinery of the law is not easily geared to making allowances for just this sort of subtlety, but it may be the psychiatrist's duty to support the mother who cannot bring herself to force this punishment on her child or to help her in pleading her case before the magistrates. Our aim is, in patient discussion, to find a plan which is fair to the child and is acceptable to each parent.

Drug-taking among teenage boys and girls is not yet a substantial problem in the age group with whom child guidance clinics mostly deal, but it may become so, and already in the remand-home population and among the adolescents who are referred for various reasons its possible existence has to be remembered. A certain amount of experimentation with the use of some less damaging drugs such as marijuana or Indian hemp, and amphetamine, among young people who are generally emotionally well adjusted, is undoubtedly going on in our midst. Although these drugs are addictive and potentially dangerous, we may have to accept a measure of this with almost as much equanimity as we have become accustomed to in the case of tobacco and alcohol. Once the matter gets beyond this playing-out stage and becomes a habit a serious situation is developing which may lead to addiction and perhaps to acquaintance with 'hard' drugs such as L.S.D. and heroin.

As part of a treatment programme we may have to consider the routine testing of urine for drugs in such places as remand homes. Diagnosis otherwise is not easy, as drug addicts are notoriously untruthful. Miller has stated that many adolescent drug-takers turn out to be highly disturbed personalities and that drug-taking is therefore not an entity.[91] Scott and Willcox consider that the problem of young amphetamine-takers is likely to resemble the problem of delinquency as a whole.[92] Connell found that all his own group of patients had problems of adolescent adjustment. He found out-patient psychotherapy to be of value and considered that there was a case for admission of some individuals to treatment units and that in other instances approved school or Borstal might best meet the young person's requirements.[93] Legislative attention to restricting sources of supply is indicated, but the present practice of issuing to addicts prescriptions for drugs *free of charge*, because they are coming for treatment, seems capable of abuse.

CHAPTER X

Introductory Considerations to Play Therapy Techniques

Children do not readily talk about their deeper problems. Sometimes they are only dimly, if at all, aware of them, and it is for these reasons that techniques for their elicitation, such as painting and play, are necessary. An inhibited, timid boy of eleven, who had been guilty of arson, depicted in colour a most realistic air battle. He was pleased with this production and to the therapist it demonstrated the existence of internal resentments and aggressions. A commonly used form of play is the sand tray, with its equipment of people, animals, motor cars, houses, trees and so forth, in which the child is encouraged to make his own 'world' or scene of his own choosing. In such tableaux of war, death, peaceful pastoral life, animal activity and so on the child depicts his own feelings and so gives leads to the intuitive or discerning doctor. Modelling, the employment of dolls' houses with their complement of inmates and furniture, and play with water, are other forms of expressive play. The importance of interpretation notwithstanding, it probably happens sometimes that without the exact nature of the problem ever coming to light the child is able to work out in play therapy his adjustment to it.

Along with the attempt to elucidate the child's problem there is a parallel quality in treatment, namely that the psychiatrist is aiming to form a friendship, more correctly a relationship, with the child. This is built upon a foundation of trying to make the child happy in the treatment room, and as a medium for this such activities as the above are useful. The child therapist whose experience is small may find it worth while to have somewhere within the child's vision simple games such as snakes and ladders or skittles, bats, skipping ropes and balls, so that the child is free to choose any of these; and helpful to talk with the child about his ordinary interests, leaving any more purposively directed play and discussion until a relationship has been established.

Verbal discussion of problems, feelings and attitudes, plays a substantial part in treatment and where appropriate the discussion of dreams is useful. Broadly speaking, the younger the child, and the more upset he is, the less he will be able to contribute in this way and the more the doctor will have to rely on his own intuition in appraising the child's contribution in play, painting or activity. Once the therapist has established a relationship with the child he can begin to interpret the child's feelings and attitudes towards *him* and from this he may help the child to develop a more healthy emotional response to his surroundings. As a rough guide, we find with children of average intelligence that once the child is about ten years of age therapy can be conducted largely at a verbal level with play or painting as ancillaries, and that our principal technique is to try to understand what the child is thinking or feeling and to help him to bring it out. Free association, as used in adult therapy, is not available from children.

What is the nuclear problem from which this child is suffering? We posed this question at the beginning of the book and it remains the enigma to be solved until we have satisfactorily answered it. As the therapist begins to grasp the answer he elucidates it in interpretation, and therapy proceeds in this way. To view the situation thus is valid whether the case requires many interviews or only one or two.

The play techniques which we employ are designed to give the therapist an opportunity to have the child project his difficulties, both his unconscious ones and those of which he is more or less aware but dare not express. Play itself can be therapeutic, but unless the child can express some feeling or accept some interpretive comment his resistances have not been overcome. At the same time the relationship he makes in play with the therapist is itself of value. Everything that the child does has some meaning in relation to his mental life – his approach to the therapist, his attitude to toys, his degree either of inhibition or of freedom, real or apparent, of self-expression, as well as what he actually does with the play material; these are all revealing to those who have eyes to see. Every impulse reflects something of unconscious fantasy. If the therapist can grasp these meanings, being assisted in doing so by all his other knowledge of the child and of his circumstances, he will thereby gain further insight into the child's emotional problem. If the therapist can interpret to the child just as much as is necessary, this shared insight will give relief to the child.

There is also the problem of the therapist's own anxieties – our inability to help, our failure to achieve a genuine rapport with the inhibited child, the times when we cannot understand what the child's inner problem is and cannot see what are the unconscious meanings of his play or behaviour – anxieties which Freud termed the counter transference. The child's resistances have to be seen as meaningful themselves. The therapist may represent to the child's unconscious a dangerous father or mother figure in relation to whom strong oedipal feelings are entertained and it will be too threatening to bring these into consciousness. Interpretation of this may be harmful and the therapist may have, instead, to support the child's ego by making a relationship with him as a friendly figure and by endeavouring to allay the strong guilt feelings that are at the core of the problem. Possibly the child may be trying out the psychiatrist; feeling that grown-ups are for ever treating him shabbily, he is going to show this adult how it feels to be denied an understanding response. The therapist's patience and his grasp of the child's need to test and to punish him may be rewarded by an eventual, greater amount of trust. If therapy is not progressing, avoid the error of rushing to the drug cupboard, of placing your faith in hypnosis or of embarking on a programme of behaviour therapy. If these remedies have been considered in the initial assessment of the case to be likely to have some value in treatment, there will be some purpose in their employment; but to introduce them because treatment is failing, unless there has been a new outlook in diagnosis which would justify a new approach, is to court even wider failure. Much better to review the child's situation anew and to consider whether one has, after all, assessed correctly what is the nuclear problem.

The frequency of interviews is relevant. If interviews were possible four of five times weekly, anxiety would be reduced and in the resulting, easier relationship defences might be relaxed. In the nature of things this is usually impossible in the average child guidance clinic and we must assume that weekly sessions will be the rule, with such relationships as can be built thereon.

Treatment in relation to emotional development: the genital phase. Of great relevance to therapy is the child's age or, rather, the stage of emotional development in which he is. Young children still in the genital phase of development will project in their play what are their emotional situations. Play releases inhibitions and disapproved impulses. The young child has few defences unless for simple denial and young children frankly express erotic material. Young children play out what their mothers want of them, in relation, for example, to toilet functions, to eating and to sleeping habits, and they show in their play what they are resisting of home discipline. Family relationships are the young child's world and these can be reproduced in play with dolls. Play is the young child's chief means of communication, but he will also verbalize within his play. The therapist attempts to build up self-confidence in the child by sharing in the friendly play atmosphere. Masturbation fantasies and fear of punishment for

PLAY THERAPY

masturbation – unconscious that is, not usually consciously recognized – are frequently of importance, as in the case of a boy who was very upset about a trivial cut on his finger. By entering into the spirit of the child's play, by listening and by friendly and sympathetic comment on the love (sex) needs of the child and on his aggressive desires, we can help him to express his feelings and his fantasies, which will thus lose some of their power to harm him. The case which follows, though of a slightly older girl, illustrates how a child's feelings may be handled in a manner that is helpful, while at the same time limiting the therapy to what is necessary.

A seven-year-old girl, Pauline, was referred to us by her doctor because of sleeping difficulties and bed-wetting and there was a history of nightmares. She was an only child of good intelligence. During pregnancy her mother had been 'very ill' with considerable loss of weight, and labour was prolonged, although there was no evidence of injury. Feeding, weaning and toilet training all presented considerable difficulties. Pauline was demanding of affection, rather than genuinely affectionate, was sensitive and had mood swings and at times she showed so obvious a preference for her father as to arouse feelings of resentment within her mother. She was destructive and at school she gave much trouble to her teachers.

Pauline came willingly into the playroom for her first interview. She was friendly and willing to talk. Of the toys in the room she chose the dolls' house, where she played happily with the dolls and furniture and she talked freely about what she was doing. In this interview she gave the impression of being a normal, happy child.

At the next interview she painted and played with a number of toys. She chatted freely much of the time and she was often demanding, asking the doctor to look at what she had done, behaviour that seemed rather more appropriate to a younger child. She was distractible, she went from one thing to another and nothing held her interest for any length of time. At the end of the interview it was difficult to persuade her to stop, a circumstance which I have come to associate with there being a sense of frustration in a child's life.

At this time we knew something of the difficulties Pauline's parents had experienced, although important details did not come to the social worker's knowledge until a later interview with her mother, who was reluctant to bring forward some of the detail. Her father ran his own shop, and although this business was successful for a time it had collapsed financially a year or two earlier and no small degree of emotional stress within the family arose from this. We also learned of an emotionally toned illness from which the mother had suffered in her early teen years and that Pauline had had one fit a year before coming to see us. Had it been decided to continue therapy in a longer number of interviews than in fact we did, more would have been discovered, but there was pretty strong evidence that Pauline's emotional needs had been to some extent neglected. This fitted in with the appearances of frustration and unconscious resentment which were revealed in the child's symptoms and in her attitude in the play situation.

At the time of the third interview Pauline's mother said to the social worker that Pauline now seemed almost well enough to stop coming. In the interview the child herself played and talked happily, no problem material emerged on this occasion and again she gave the impression of a normal child. We discussed the question of stopping treatment soon; she wished to continue for a little longer and she then agreed to the therapist's suggestion of two more visits.

In the last interview Pauline talked naturally. She went to the lavatory and on her return she pulled up her frock to show the doctor her slip and showed him the doll's pants. He asked about wanting to be a boy and to have a 'wee-wee'. She said when she wanted to be a boy it was because she wanted to fight; not to have a 'wee-wee', but to be a boy with a girl's body. When he asked if she were sleeping better she said she read herself a few stories and thus could go to sleep. Then she told him of the family's plans for a new home. She next said that she objected to her mother and father bringing strange people into her bedroom, as it was rude for them to see her if she had no upper part to her pyjamas. It would have been interesting to have followed these sexual fantasies in subsequent interviews. It was probably sufficient for her immediate needs that they had been mentioned and had been accepted by the therapist. Pauline appeared to have achieved a satisfactory degree of adjustment and he deemed it appropriate to stand by the decision to terminate therapy at this session.

Inhibition or shyness is one of the attitudes we most commonly encounter. Somehow we have to help this child to feel at home and this will mean forgetting all about the symptoms for the time being. Part of the work of therapy is to make the child happy and the gulf between him and the stranger who is the therapist has to be bridged. Here, then, is a frightened child or an extremely self-conscious girl or boy whom the therapist has to entertain. In doing this we shall remember roughly what is his age and his intelligence level; we may begin with the sand tray, we may offer toys, dolls or model cars or paper and paints, the blackboard or chalk or boats to sail in the basin. These are offered to the child almost as one offers eatables at a tea party, and the therapist may also offer to take part in the play.

One's form of presentation of the various available choices is peculiar to the individual therapist. One says one has got this and that, shows them, shows how to play with them, asks the child if he will join in with the therapist at, for example, pushing a model car across the floor and, indeed, devotes oneself for the present simply to being nice to the child. With children who are over the age of eight or ten and who are too inhibited, even with encouragement, to make a scene on the sand or to paint, a doll or a ball may appeal, but it may be equally profitable to try to talk, humanly and naturally, about things that are real to the child and yet not too emotional. 'Do tell me a little about yourself. I wonder if you have a dog at home or a pussy? I think you go to All Saints' School. What do you like best at school? Tell me what you don't like.' I ask about the teachers, I ask if he has friends at school and I ask about enemies, explaining that by this last term I mean the sort of people who tease you or annoy you. It is sufficient for the moment if we can find some form of conversation or some kind of play that will give the child interest or pleasure.

Sometimes the therapist cannot persuade the child to come into the playroom without his mother. Such a child will always agree to come if the mother comes, too, and rather than frighten the child it is better to have them both. In the room one tries to get the child to take part in some play activity with mother as an onlooker. Often she will be able to leave during the interview and one gets the child alone, but just occasionally this privilege has to be postponed to a later visit. It is worth remembering that the purpose of having the child alone with the therapist is in order to make a relationship with him, wherein he will be able to say or to do things that he would be inhibited or prevented from doing if his mother or someone else were present also, and the achievement of this relationship will not be facilitated by rushing things or by anything which frightens or alienates him at the beginning. Consideration for the child's feelings and an attempt to understand his immediate situation at the present moment, as well as the circumstances of the problem for which he is referred, and *respect* for these feelings, are paramount, especially at this early stage of treatment.

Treatment in the latency phase. The unconscious emotions of children in this phase are hidden behind the strongest of defences. Love and sex responses are repressed, imagination is limited and the child confronts us with an attitude of reserve and distrust. The ego is not fully developed, they do not know that they are ill and they have no desire to be cured. They have great difficulty in speaking of their feelings for their parents. A child, however, who is regressed may display qualities more appropriate to the genital phase. The play of latency children is more structured, is more symbolic, has more elaborate schemes of interpersonal relationship and is less easy to interpret. Play, nevertheless, is the portal to conversation and provides the opening gambit of contact between therapist and child. The other important factor is transference. Were it not for transference the child would withdraw from relevant communication with the therapist. Play and the therapist's attitudes of understanding and sympathy provide the foundation for a relationship in which everyday problems, and eventually, perhaps, some deeper ones, can be discussed.

Therapy which involves insight is, for these reasons, swimming against the stream of natural development at this phase; it is therefore likely to be unsuccessful and may do harm. Treatment which attempts to strengthen the personality rather than to penetrate defences is going along with the flow of development, is less difficult to undertake and may give better promise of results. This does not mean that the psychiatrist can let up in his efforts himself to gain insight into the nature of the child's problem. In dealing with latency children we must accept that any speaking on their part will deal with topics that are 'acceptable' and that they will seldom verbalize anything of their real feelings. How far we should try to interpret is a matter for delicate decision, but it will be wise to allow that the child will have secrets that he prefers to keep to himself and we should be wary of violating this privilege. The achievement of a limited objective in therapy during latency will be of greater value than a struggle to lay bare the emotions, which ends in the stalemate of a no-man's-land between the therapist and the patient.

With many children in this age group our best work will lie in the area of integrating the unity of child and family. To enable the parents better to understand the child and, equally important, to enable them to become more aware of the nature of their own reactions towards him – to achieve this may be our most important contribution to therapy.

Treatment in adolescence. The adolescent combines the need to exteriorize his sexual instincts, which is reminiscent of the young child's lack of inhibition, with the reserve that is characteristic of the latency child. Unconscious sexual guilt is a powerful inhibiting factor and the conflict between this and his sexual desires produces no small emotional stress even in an adolescent who is not emotionally ill. His relationships are disturbed by conflicting needs and there is great pressure to escape from the guilt-provoking authority of adults. Hence there will usually be strong resistance to the emergence of emotion during therapy. Unlike the case in children, we may expect an adolescent who is aware of his need of psychological help to be capable of free association, but we shall be so fortunate only infrequently. Winnicott has said that the cure of adolescent problems is the passage of time.

Broadly speaking the adolescent's problems will lie in the field of sex awareness and sexual need, in disturbed relationships with his parents and in the difficulties he finds in making relationships with others of his own, as well as of the opposite, sex. It will usually be as much as we can do and therefore all that we need attempt, if we assess what the principal problems are with which the boy or girl is contending, and if we aim, through a therapy of relationship and insight, to deal with these. Winnicott has also suggested that treatment for adolescents should be given, 'on demand so to speak', the adolescent being invited to choose when and how often he or she wishes to come. Occasionally we meet the adolescent who wishes (and therefore needs) treatment at short intervals over a long period of time, and there is also an impression, borne of experience, that if there is to be treatment *at depth* during adolescence it is likely to have to be continued in some degree throughout this stage of development.

A difficulty arises in the case of delinquency or severe behaviour disorder. These persons, usually boys, have no small problem, but more often than not they are unwilling to discuss it, and the therapist is left with the uphill task of making a relationship with a recalcitrant youth, for it is only on the basis of rapport between patient and therapist that emotional problems can be discussed with any meaning. A further difficulty sometimes faces the male therapist when dealing with adolescent girls in that their inhibition against talking of sexual matters with a man may be almost insurmountable. This will arise especially in families where sexual morality is loose, for it is among them that the guilt sense is strongest and the therapist is seen as avenging and menacing. Occasionally, too, when sexual issues have arisen, one runs into difficulty on account of religious scruple, especially with families of the Catholic faith, and the therapist would be unwise if he did not pay regard to these resistances.

On the other hand, to the therapist who has been struggling with the issues of the latency period it may come as a relief that his next patient is an adolescent. By and large, adolescent patients do co-operate, and although the technique of free association is still not one that we can freely employ, they generally display a readiness to talk about their problems, a feature which is so often lacking in the younger child. In therapy one has to be prepared to go a long way with the adolescent, to grasp that his point of view, even if socially unacceptable, is a reasonable one as viewed through the teenage eye, and to accept that the criticisms he makes of other, and usually older, persons – parents and teachers, for example – are not without validity. This, of course, is not to say that one must agree with all that these youths and girls say, but it is imperative that we should have a healthy respect for their viewpoints even if these are not rational in the light of all the evidence or if they appear dangerous, recognizing that these beliefs cannot be altered by argument. They can be discussed in a permissive manner, however, and in an explanatory way we may illustrate the difficulties with which those who are being criticized are having to contend. It is essential that the relationship is one in which the young person feels that his ideas are accepted and that there is no possibility of ridicule in the therapist's response to whatever he may do or say or reveal. The relationship must be one in which he can feel safe because the therapist is, so far as is humanly possible, totally understanding, has the young person's immediate interests – not just his long-term ones – completely at heart, and is not secretly in league with any authoritative system or concept. It will sometimes be appropriate to manipulate adult attitudes within the entourage.

CHAPTER XI

Techniques of Play Therapy

The sand tray. Margaret Lowenfeld is the greatest exponent of the use of the sand tray and she has found it to be a valuable projection technique from childhood up well into the teens. Older children, in many cases, consider it too unsophisticated for their 'mature' years, and if the device is to be used with older children it will probably be necessary to get their co-operation to the extent that they know they are using the sand tray to depict their own situations in life. Soddy has warned that with children above the age of about eight or ten there is a risk that the child will employ the sand tray as an escape mechanism whereby he can play in the sand, use up time and thus avoid having to face up to reality in his interviews with the therapist.

It is worth while going to a certain amount of trouble to get hold of a fair selection of sand-tray toys. Animals, motor cars, toy soldiers and 'cowboys' are easy to come by, but it is more difficult to find a selection of ordinary people. Among animals the tortoise is traditionally associated with safety and the snake with either sex or healing, and this latter reptile was most difficult to obtain in form suitable for the sand tray, until I at last discovered a specimen in 'Gamages'. Houses, trees, hedges, gates, a little boat and such other everyday objects as one can think of or see in the toyshop complete the set. It is useful to have a box divided into at least four compartments, so that the child can easily select one type of piece from another.

Lowenfeld regards the sand tray as the child's 'world' – it is his place and he can make his own world in it. Personally I find the concept of 'world' rather ambitious and I say to the boy or girl something like this. 'This sand is just anywhere. It's your own town or your own country, just anywhere you like. What I'd like you to do is just to make your own place in it – just whatever you like. There are these trees and houses and people and the other things. This is a house (and I put one in the sand) and this is a tree. I'll leave you for a little while to make just what you like.' In any subsequent interview it is simply a case of agreeing with the child that he make a scene in the sand tray.

In the first interview it is instructive to notice how the child approaches and applies himself to the task. Most children easily take to it, but occasionally we meet the child who is so anxious or inhibited that he merely stands and looks. Even with encouragement to make any kind of place he likes with these people, animals or trees, he may still remain too afraid. In these instances I find something else for him to do – perhaps he will paint, or he may play with bricks, or it may be that the interview has achieved as much as is possible in a single day, in which event I say that perhaps he would like to come back to see if we can find Mummy. To arrange a private chat with his mother may now be equally difficult, as he will not leave her, but with the help of the social worker or the secretary it may be possible to do this.

From his manner of approach we get an idea of the child's degree of self-confidence and from the way he employs the pieces in making his sand scene we discover something of his capacity to express his emotions; from the form the scene takes we learn about his predominant characteristics, such as love-seeking or aggression, and from the actual structure of the scene we may gain knowledge of the problem from which he suffers, particularly if he is willing to tell us the story of the scene that is depicted. We can now take these features separately.

The average child will purposefully tackle the task of producing a sand scene and will display some confidence in choosing and placing the pieces. The inhibited child is slow and diffident and may need encouragement to take even this amount of independent action, and this child is likely to need a great deal of understanding support from his environment before he can stand on his own feet.

Brighter children usually have no difficulty in finding a theme, although an inhibited, bright child may have the intellectual capacity, but be unable to express his feelings, so that he will produce a poor tableau. Duller children and those whose capacity for expression is poor may set out the pieces in the sand at random, in straight lines all facing the same way, or may even set out every one of the pieces without the resultant scene having any meaning. Such children are unlikely to be lacking in imagination so much as in need of help in bringing it out.

It is useful to distinguish between introverted and extraverted children. The child who is introverted may express much in small compass: a soldier may represent an army or a wild animal a host of evil forces seeking to dominate the individual, whereas the extravert will more expansively try to express the wealth of his feelings through a corresponding expenditure of sand-tray toys.

Two forms of sand scene are particularly common. One of these is the farm type of scene, and this is usually produced by the anxious, inhibited child whose great need seems to be for security and support. There are variations: the animals may enjoy a measure of freedom to roam about or they may be closely penned in, according to the child's view of what life is or ought to be. The farm may be protected against marauding 'Indians' or may be threatened by wild animals or the whole atmosphere may be one of peaceful and protected existence. These forms of expression have to be interpreted against the background of oedipal anxieties, the child's fear of his own power to harm others and his concern, perhaps at a more conscious level, of the threat which those in his immediate environment represent to him. In the initial interview it is probably sufficient to store such ideas in our own minds. In later interviews we may be able to collate such impressions with what we know of the child's problem from other sources, and in our conversation with him to bring out anxieties of which he finds it difficult to speak.

The second common form of scene is the battleground. This may be of the 'Cowboy and Indian' type or it may be of opposing armies. Ideas culled from television programmes naturally exert their influence and the idea of the Germans as our traditional enemy unfortunately lives on in the minds of many youngsters who were still unborn long after hostilities ceased. These warlike scenes probably represent a healthy expression of aggressive instinct, and although it will sometimes be appropriate to achieve verbal exteriorization of the child's hatreds, I believe it will often be equally beneficial to let well alone.

Returning to the very anxious children, we usually find in later interviews that the ice is partly broken and that the sand tray is accepted. We already have discovered something of the child's fear of separation from his mother in a strange setting, so that the therapist must become, if possible, one of his loved objects. To do this one does not want to lose sight of the problem for which the child has been brought, and in a sense the child is interested in this as a problem, yet the more immediate need is to reveal an interest in the child's desires of the moment. Too often the most obvious of these desires is that the therapist should keep off the subject-matter of the problem. Even if this demand ought largely to be met, it is a good plan that somewhere in each interview interpretive comment that is relevant to the problem should be brought in. From a study of the child's play in the sand tray, with toys or directly with the therapist, the therapist should derive some relevant meaning, even if it is only to indicate the child's fear of not being loved or of being rejected.

It is probably better to allow Mummy to be in the room or to let the child go to her if he is anxious and wishes to do so, until such time as he feels sufficiently secure to remain willingly alone with the therapist. The male therapist may be at a disadvantage with some of these timid children who are naturally more apprehensive of father figures than of mother figures, but often this can be overcome through understanding and patience. Once matters of a preliminary kind have been dealt with, it is a good rule to avoid asking questions so far as this is possible. Emotionally toned questions are a challenge to the child, an attack from which he is often forced to recoil in silence or in replies that have no bearing on the truth. Instead one tries to be imaginatively insightful and to play back, as it were, to the child the record of his thoughts.

The theory behind most work with the sand tray is, of course, that the child will project his emotions, including those not ordinarily allowed into consciousness, in the scenes he makes. There are also such subsidiary values as that sand play is enjoyable to the child and that it can provide a talking point with him. It has not, however, been the experience of all child therapists that the sand tray is of *great* usefulness. It is a convenient technique for studying the child in the first interview, but I have found it to be of more limited value in later interviews and certainly less generally useful than painting. Probably the idiosyncrasies of the therapist, as much as the needs of the child, will be the deciding factor as to whether the sand tray is going to be employed as a major or only as an occasional form of therapy.

A ten-year-old girl of average intelligence was referred to the clinic because of anxiety and unhappiness. The problem had begun suddenly as being afraid to go to school and unwilling to leave her mother. We were in the fortunate position of knowing a good deal about this family already, as we had treated an older brother some years previously, and we were aware that the father had been in and out of mental hospital and prison and that there had been a divorce.

In my first interview with Ellen I suggested a sand scene. She constructed in the sand two farms, one of which had been destroyed in a tremendous storm. A crocodile was hiding in his den far away at the other side of the sand tray. He was the cause of the storm, which had, indeed, not only destroyed the one farm but had slightly damaged the other. An ostrich had escaped from the first farm to the second.

Bearing father's behaviour in mind, it seemed that he might well be the crocodile and Ellen the ostrich, who had 'escaped' from the original (destroyed) home of the days before her father broke it up to the new home of the time following his being divorced. On this assumption I asked her if the crocodile were bad (to have caused so much damage) or if he were good inside. She said he was good inside,

PLAY TECHNIQUES

that some of his family had died and that it had made him like that. She was worried that he was cold and lonely. The real problem was the loss and 'badness' of her father, whom she loved and about whom she could not avoid having ambivalent feelings. On this premiss she was taken for treatment in the clinic.

At one point in a subsequent sand scene a number of people and animals were hunting the crocodile and the therapist afterwards said that this meant that Ellen wanted to punish Daddy for deserting her, but that she also very much wanted him to come back. This sort of play, interpretation and discussion may seem, in fact, to alter nothing. What it does is to bring into the open the child's unspoken feelings, to make a visible (or audible) issue of anxieties that have not been fully conscious and which, therefore, the child has been unable to handle rationally, and to provide an opportunity for sharing these anxieties with the therapist.

I believe that some children who are depressed are in that state because of anxieties which, though not entirely unconscious, are submerged into the subconscious strata of feeling, and that this displays itself, as depressions do, by a demeanour of sadness, by some degree of retardation and sometimes by behaviour disorder. This, I believe, is occasionally the reason why a child steals. I believe that, by contrast, anxieties of which the child is fully conscious cause sadness, but that the child has a better understanding of why he is sad and that the sadness is periodic because at times other matters are uppermost in his mind, so that he is happy. If the anxieties causing depression can be contemplated and shared, the child has thereby a better chance to manipulate his situation and so, with the help of the love relationships he enjoys, to achieve recovery. Such was the rationale of Ellen's treatment. It appeared to produce an improvement in her condition and this limited gain was regarded as worth while in relation to the time that had been spent on therapy.

Derek was referred at the age of seven and a half on account of anxiety, stammer, enuresis, crying easily and a number of psychosomatic symptoms. His I.Q. was 112. His mother was an anxious individual who had been in a mental hospital for a month when he was a baby, his father was a quiet man, fond of his children, and there was one younger sister. These circumstances, plus a possible constitutional loading, were regarded as having contributed largely to the boy's nervousness.

Derek's treatment consisted of a series of paintings, sand scenes and a good deal of imaginative and mildly interpretive talk on the therapist's part. We shall largely confine ourselves to his sand scenes. In the first of these he made a farm, separated by a fence from an area occupied by Red Indians. He said that they were fighting. (By this time we had already had one or two paintings depicting aggressive features and it had been largely agreed between us that one part of this timid boy did, indeed, want to fight.) In the case of the painting we discussed the fighting aspect and in time he told of a boy, Crowhurst, who annoyed him. He said that Crowhurst swore and he did not, and the therapist suggested that perhaps the reason why this bothered him was that Crowhurst could say angry things when he felt like it, but Derek could not. Derek said he never felt angry. This was the fourth interview and the therapist wondered if this intelligent child was already under too much super-ego pressure to allow of his exteriorizing his feelings for the time being. A discussion with the social worker at this juncture elicited her opinion to the effect that there was little hope of the parents becoming more permissive of his developing an independent personality than at the time they were. In the next session he arrived too tidily dressed and wearing a bow tie. He painted a pirate ship and admitted some desire to be a pirate.

Several interviews passed before his next sand scene and in one of these he mentioned his inability to get to sleep at night, with the result that he was able to say a little of his feelings about his parents' restrictiveness and about his school difficulties. The sand scene on this occasion was of an army in readiness to fight. In the next interview he brought a compass. He liked this little instrument, but the interesting feature is the symbolism whereby it represents a guide to finding his way in life which was just what we were attempting to do in the psychotherapeutic sessions.

His next sand scene was of horsemen and archers fighting. The therapist referred to his need to fight, his hating people who got the better of him and yet being afraid to retaliate. He also said that sometimes he must wish he could fight his father or at least be as strong as he and able to stand up to him. Derek, in a whisper, admitted some truth in most of this, but the therapist was left with the feeling that he was barely getting through to him. In the following session he painted the bombing of an armoured car and his association to this was that he would be lying down on the ground, trying to escape. The therapist asked if he felt threatened. Derek said he did, but could not say why. They continued to talk about this and he said he felt like being chased. By everyone, the therapist suggested, and he said this was so. Asked why, he said it might be for spying on his enemies.

Some weeks earlier the therapist had felt that it could be beneficial to open up the sexual subject a little, and the boy's use of the word 'spying' in relation to himself provided an opportunity. The therapist said that he thought there was another kind of spying – spying on girls in the toilet, in the bathroom and so forth. Derek said 'No' to this, but the therapist replied: 'I wonder.' He went on to say that there was also curiosity about babies, how they grew inside their mummies, and how they were born, and of this Derek was slightly more accepting.

In his next sand scene soldiers had captured Indians and had killed animals which had come in to eat the Indians. He himself was second-in-command of the soldiers. Who was in command? All the therapist could get here was that he preferred his father to his mother because his father could help him to make things. He then named a boy who had hit him with an anorak and he agreed with the therapist that he would have liked to put his sword into the boy's throat as, in the sand scene, the soldier had done to the crocodile. I believe that to bring out aggression in this manner will have a safety-valve effect and that it will counter rather than enhance the opposite tendency, which would be to carry out anti-social acts.

Two weeks after the crocodile sand scene Derek appeared to be a good deal better, although he still occasionally had psychosomatic symptoms. He was by this time able to talk more naturally in his interviews than had been the case earlier on; the therapist felt that he might very soon be able to carry on under his own steam and after discussing the matter with him it was agreed that he come once more. The alternative would have been to continue batting for a long time on a wicket so sticky that results could hardly be commensurate with the amount of time spent.

At the last interview he made a further sand scene in which there was a good deal of close fighting and in which a crocodile took a prominent part. Derek agreed with the therapist that one part of him would like to be taking part in this fighting. The therapist suggested that the crocodile's name was 'Crowhurst'. Concurrently with this interview Derek's mother was seeing the social worker and the possibility was left open for her to see the social worker sometimes even though the boy's interviews had ceased. She told the social worker that Derek no longer was stammering, but that he still sometimes soiled his underpants, and she wept because the interviews were to cease.

Six months afterwards Derek's mother had several weeks as an inpatient in a neurosis centre because of an access of sub-acute anxiety. Some eight months after her return home she continued to complain of Derek's behaviour, but his father considered that she was being overanxious regarding this. Few cases have better illustrated the total family nature of a problem which has initially presented as a series of neurotic symptoms in a child.

Water has its place in the sand tray. Water has an elemental quality and its employment can provide freedom of expression for a variety of emotions even if these are not individually capable of being interpreted. It is not necessary that the therapist should understand just what each of the child's performances mean.

Play with toys and materials. The range of toys available in the clinic, while obviously not the most important adjunct to success, is none the less of some significance, and the less-experienced therapist can make life just that much easier for himself and more enjoyable for his patients by having a well-equipped playroom. A whole afternoon spent in the toyshops, provided it is a rare event, may not be the least service that the therapist does for his patients, and he who cannot face this may find that his social worker, or even his wife, will do it for him, provided he is prepared to give a careful brief of the kind of things that are wanted.

Structured toys, those that have to be manipulated in a certain way, constructional toys and those that by their nature give the child a set piece to perform, as well as games of this type, tend to be an embarrassment, as they positively encourage the child to escape into a play world where the answer is provided for him, so to speak, with the result that expression of his own instincts can be withheld. With this proviso a fair variety is an advantage, though the playroom should not represent such a plethora of playthings as to be distracting. A couple of games of the draughts and snakes and ladders type are occasionally useful in paving the way to a relationship with an apprehensive child. It is probably better for the therapist not to suggest such a game, but to have the games somewhere where the child may see them. The same applies with toys generally, that they should be easily accessible to the child, who will usually be given a free choice in what he wishes to do.

A dolls' house with furniture, and not forgetting kitchen and bathroom furniture, is useful, and there should be a family of dolls, suitable in size to inhabit the house. A few dolls of ordinary size, and if possible representing both sexes, are a valuable asset. There is room for ingenuity in selecting materials, but the following at least are suggested: cars, train, a gun, boats and aeroplanes, blocks of wood for instinctive building, a ball, Plasticine or clay, paper and scissors and one or two imaginative odds and ends. A blackboard and chalks are valuable, the blackboard preferably fixed to the wall, but I have not found crayons of much value unless it is impossible in some emergency to get paints. A pencil and rubber are always useful. A sink, fixed at suitably low level, gives scope for play with boats and other water play and provides a source of water for those children who wish to use water with the sand tray. Children sometimes ask for special materials, such as wood and nails and in one of my clinics I have obtained these along with the necessary tools.

The therapist's part in the play may be stated as to watch interestedly, even encouragingly at times, and to try to comprehend what the play signifies. The child may play out, with dolls, for example, the treatment he receives at home, like the little girl who was 'mother' in her play and criticized, scolded and slapped her dolls. (We knew this child's mother as demanding, frustrated and impatient: her daughter's play illustrated how intolerant she could be as well.) He may play out his parents' wishes for good behaviour, conforming or tidiness, or he may reveal deeper anxieties, as Sheila who enacted cruel scenes in the dolls' house. He may play out his own wishes and emotional needs, punishing the doll who represents the envied sibling, or the figure who stands for father or mother who is loved or hated, according to circumstances. His play may be rebellious or destructive, scattering toys or splashing water around in the sand tray – an exteriorization of the hatred unconsciously felt against introjected prohibiting parental figures. In one of our clinics my room used to be heated by a coal fire, since replaced in the interests of smoke abatement by a more impersonal electric heater, and a rejected little boy used at each interview to remove one by one with the tongs, the burning coals and spread them on the grate below. The significance of this was not clear, but he felt unloved and his destruction of our source of warmth was perhaps a dramatization of this. The child's presenting symptom was that he systematically made large cuts in his clothes with scissors. It is unlikely to be meaningful to the child if one interprets this sort of thing directly, but it is relevant to say 'You feel I don't love you and you will punish me by making the room cold the way you feel cold and you feel that people aren't friendly.' Interpretation of a doll's behaviour in play may be accepted, where if applied to the child in real life it would be denied.

A critical difficulty in therapy with children is the child's unconscious fear of the therapist. The degree of this fear is influenced by a number of factors, but the essential matter is sexual guilt which will usually have stemmed mainly from the unconscious emotional experiences of the oedipal phase. The therapist is seen in fantasy as a disapproving, punishing figure, the representative of the unconscious picture of the parents who will destroy the child because of his oedipal desires and jealousies, the castrating parent who will mutilate him because of his sensual wishes. Thus the unconscious feeling the child has is that the therapist is dangerous. A girl in treatment said that she was afraid the therapist might get angry and shout at her.

TREATMENT FOR CHILDREN

Actually these children feel that the therapist, however kindly to the conscious reasoning, would be intensely rejecting and damning of the child's impulses – loving, sensual, aggressive or acquisitive – if he knew what these were. To see the therapist as another human being who must, therefore, have the same sexual needs and excretory functions as the patient has himself, is something which the child's unconscious guilt feelings simply cannot allow. Obviously this will apply with much greater force in some children than in others, and as a matter of experience, where delinquent behaviour is the problem or where sexual difficulties are at issue, these resistances are at their strongest. This helps to explain why many children cannot talk to the therapist or cannot even accept interpretations. Sometimes it is worth while to interpret to the child how he does feel this way about oneself, although in doing so one has to avoid postulating to the child desires, hatreds or jealousies which it would be too traumatic for him to allow to enter his consciousness.

Play techniques of one or two special kinds exist, such as modelling with clay, Plasticine or the like. Clay particularly has the delightful quality of being messy, malleable, wet and sticky, and unconsciously reminiscent of faeces. Some children are more likely to be at home in modelling than are others and their productions will provide material for understanding their instinctual needs and for interpretation, but it seems to me that the aptitudes of the therapist are relevant here and I have not myself used the method widely. As with other forms of play therapy, the therapist needs to be attentive to and interested in the child's play. Sometimes the child will wish the therapist to take a direct hand in the play and when this happens it usually is right to do so.

Play situations are another special technique.[94] These also seem to call for special aptitude on the doctor's part and are open to the objection that the child is being given a set piece and that he is therefore likely to 'smell a rat', and to colour his response accordingly. Toys used are a mother doll, father doll, self doll (representing the patient), brother, sister and baby dolls and a peer doll (representing another child such as a playmate). The therapist conjures up a situation known or likely to have been encountered by the child in real life, sets the appropriate dolls in this situation and asks the child to carry on with the play. He may, for instance, sit the mother doll down, suckling the baby, bring the self doll beside them, and say: 'This boy has just run in to ask his Mummy for a drink. He finds that she cannot give it to him just now because she is feeding baby. Can you show me what happens next?' To structure these situations will provide the doctor with opportunities to use his imagination. Situations involving

PLAY TECHNIQUES

separation anxieties, sexual curiosity, intercourse fantasies in the parents' bedroom, rivalry between siblings, interpersonal stresses with mates at school, parental aggression or punishment, or the eerie drabness of coming home after school in winter to a house which is empty because mother is out at work – these and others will lend themselves to representation in this manner. If the child puts feeling into his response something will be achieved. If occasion were to warrant it, breasts or genital organs for a doll could be fashioned from Plasticine, provided the therapist bore in mind that it is the emotional fantasies pertaining to sex that are relevant, rather than the anatomical features. Specific threats to which the child has been exposed can be re-enacted using the dolls. Conflict situations may similarly be presented in dramatic form.

A baby's bottle with teat is a useful thing to have in the playroom and in the setting of security which the therapeutic interview provides some children will suck the bottle and may derive gain from being able to do so in the doctor's presence. A boy of eleven started the interview by telling the therapist that the baby had been born and was a girl. He soon commenced to handle the baby's bottles standing on the clinic shelf and he asked the therapist if children sometimes played with them. The therapist replied that one was actually doing so now. It took the boy some moments to tumble to the significance of this remark, but when he did he smiled. The therapist said that he might like to be a baby at the bottle himself and the boy said quite firmly that he would. This boy had come to us because of psychosomatic abdominal pain and the emotions which this sort of symptom signifies were now being portrayed in his play.

Balloon bursting is said to be useful in encouraging self-assertion in inhibited children, and the best way to do this may be to tie the balloon on the water tap and let the child turn on the water. In one of our clinics we have a punch ball which may serve a similar end and which is regarded as an outlet for aggression. When treating children in a group I have sometimes employed *drama*, getting the children to act out such a scene as the following. The family are seated together at supper when the policeman calls to inform the parents that Billy has been stealing. The children are expected to make the going once the therapist has outlined the plot.

Puppetry is a challenging technique both of self-expression and of emotional projection, providing to the child opportunities for abreaction and to the therapist for initiative. Bryan, working in Liverpool, developed it as his principal technique of therapy.[95] To witness Bryan's work was impressive, but the main drawback to the extensive use of the system is that few will have the skill and industry which

Bryan has displayed in the construction of about seventy puppets to represent every imaginable type of human figure and a few ancillaries such as witches and animals into the bargain. There seems to be no other way of obtaining the desirable repertory of pieces, although the method is open to anyone to use who has the necessary initiative and imaginative capacity.

The 'theatre' is so constructed that both the child and the therapist can play parts and the child is invited to choose whichever part (and appropriate puppet) he wishes to play and to select whom he would like the therapist's puppet to impersonate. At other times the therapist, on the basis of his knowledge of the child's past circumstances, will stage a scene along with the child in which the puppets represent the original actors. Fears and phobias are dealt with by the use of nightmarish puppets, ghosts, devils and so on, who frighten the puppet representing the child. Figures representing illness or death, sexual assault, violence and the 'dear octopus' figure with a loving face and constrictive tentacles, guilt figures representing the pointing figure of conscience and the beckoning figure of the law have their obvious uses. Bryan has found puppetry valuable both in diagnosis, where the child will act out and even verbalize what he would not say in ordinary conversation, and in therapy, where the acting out has brought the anxiety into the open and allowed it to be dealt with.

CHAPTER XII

Painting and Blackboard Drawing

Paintings are the therapeutic tool that I have found to be, on the whole, more useful than any other. The method has the disadvantage of being only two-dimensional, but against that is the unlimited variety of scene which can be depicted. If the child has elected to paint, or I have invited him to do so, I ask him to paint anything he likes, not anything he sees in the room, but something just from himself. Some workers give a lead sometimes to the child, but as far as I ever go myself is to suggest, exceptionally, that the child might paint something bad.

The attitude with which the child approaches his painting is important. Most children will easily start to paint. The most inhibited will sit, motionless and miserable, in front of the paper, and in their case one has to be encouraging. Sometimes I suggest the child almost let the brush paint whatever it likes. At times the 'butterfly' is a useful demonstration to the child of what can be done. One simply makes some dabs and strokes of wet paint on one half of the paper and then folds the two halves together. The result is usually a pretty mixture of colours. Obsessional or controlled children sometimes want to draw the outline first, in pencil. Naturally one agrees to this if the child so desires. Such behaviour indicates the child's fear of free exteriorization of himself, and it may be useful at a later time to interpret to him that this is so, and that he evidently is too afraid of criticism of anything that he may produce. There are timid children who are afraid to paint anything in case it is not good enough and there are those who, from fear or dislike, just say that they cannot paint or do not want to. This, too, it is best to accept, but perhaps in the hope that once the child is a shade more confident in the therapist he will paint. There is the cautious child who merely draws instead, either because he is obsessionally exact or else because he is afraid to let himself go in the free expression that straight painting implies. Some obsessional children characterize their paintings by having to cover the whole page completely.

Where painting is out one has to offer some other kind of play. In a recent instance of a girl who would not paint it turned out that she was interested in cookery and in needlework, and most of the interview was spent in talking about these pursuits by way of establishing rapport with her.

The general character of the painting can teach us a good deal when considered in relation to the history. A schoolboy,[96] keen on Rugby football, painted a booted foot kicking the ball. Such bland paintings are not of much help to us, as they avoid areas of anxiety, although this was of some interest as an expression of aggression (kicking) in a boy who stammered and of whose usual behaviour one would have said that butter would not melt in his mouth. Sometimes a child paints a pattern which consists merely of dividing the paper into sections of different colours. This, again, is an escape method. An intelligent but anxious and insecure boy collected butterflies as his hobby and time after time in the clinic he painted butterflies and added their names to the illustrations. Unless as a limited talking point and as something to give him pleasure in the early interviews, this work had little therapeutic value. Several months elapsed before he painted anything else, when one day he produced a galleon with shells exploding in the sea around it and a fire on the afterdeck. This revealed underlying aggression, an interpretation borne out by angry behaviour at home a year or two later. In the meantime, when he did not paint, most of our time had been spent in conversation in which the therapist's imaginative capacities were taxed to their limit.

A boy of five years and nine months was referred by his family doctor. He was an unhappy child who earlier had had infantile eczema. He also suffered from asthma, he occasionally wet his bed and was described as being spiteful and unable to fit into the family unit. He was the fourth child in a family of five. The psychologist regarded him as being of average ability, but he was too inhibited to co-operate in the test and he was not able to say a word in his interviews either with her or with the psychiatrist. His father was intolerant and refused to come to see us in the clinic, but his mother was rated as kindly.

This child painted a picture which was a great wash of black over three-quarters of the page. The remaining quarter was a large, round area of dark green on top of the black, with just a little bit of blue over the black at the foot of the page. This he did for the psychiatrist in the initial interview, so that it was his only positive contribution and it clearly portrayed his unhappy state. He was treated by a lady therapist who was with us only temporarily and had to leave after the thirteenth session. Nevertheless he was happier when seen almost ten months after his first visit, and he had had no asthma for about four months, although he was still restless and aggressive.

PAINTING

The commonest form of painting, especially from girls, is a house. All sorts of things can be imagined into this, depending on the amount of light and darkness, the size of the windows, the chimney or the amount of detail generally. Enquiry may elicit that it is the child's own home or it may be some other that is envied or is idealized. The house may be happy, warm and comforting or it may be dark and uninviting, and from these characteristics we may derive understanding of the child's emotional needs. More often than not the indication is a need to be secure, to have love and to be able to love. Without going so far as to postulate a desire to re-enter the womb, which to me always seemed a slightly far-fetched preoccupation even for the unconscious, one can often see in these paintings longings to return to the loved and cared-for state of babyhood. In talking to such a girl or boy we can say that one part of him still has such longings. This is often accepted when it becomes possible to discuss the rewards and joys of growing up into a wider, more independent life, as against the inner desire to remain in the safe love of the cradle. His present-day difficulties, the sibling jealousy which torments him, the rejection he experiences at home, the bullying and teasing at school or the menace of authority everywhere – these are factors which it may be possible to unfold with him gently and gradually. Sometimes the therapist is at a loss how to answer the child's question as to how he can handle these immediate threats which seem beyond his power to cope with. It is probable that to be able to discuss these issues with the therapist, who understands and gives moral support, is more important than any words that are used. One has to remember that, after all, unless in those cases where the child is currently being subjected to real rejection or actual cruelty, the ultimate problem is an internal one. It is the inner feeling of inferiority which disables the child from taking his siblings in his stride or from handling the teasings of his schoolfellows or the severity of his teachers in such a way that they will not reduce him to unhappiness.

Important as these considerations are, what usually interests us most in a painting is its detail. A simple picture was that of a nine-year-old girl who had been referred because of outbursts of aggressive behaviour and because she was unhappy. A street ran diagonally across the page, there were three houses with gardens and trees on one side and on the other a single house and a number of fields. In the street was a single car, in one of the fields two sheep and behind the single house was a girl in blue frock and red apron. A country village with a solitary girl was the obvious interpretation and it fitted well the child's emotional state. Yet it was a picture of an attractive setting, the sheep suggest food and clothes, the car is a lifeline with the outer world, the girl's bright colours indicated at least traces of joy in her personality and the total goodness of the picture held promise of basically warm relationships in the child's home. We did, in fact, see direct evidence of her warmth for father when he brought her to the clinic, while the fact of her nother's being in a mental hospital did not diminish the accuracy with which this picture represented the child's feelings.

A twelve-year-old girl of good intelligence came to us after a long period of anxiety-motivated school refusal. Early in her treatment she painted three identical girls, dressed in black, with black hair, red eyes, nose and mouth and white stockings. The background to this was a criss-crossing of red paint all over the page. She could say little about these girls and this is a common experience with children that they can tell us almost nothing about what they paint. Thus the therapist has usually to make his own deductions and to employ these insights with discretion in speaking to his patient. Only two colours, apart from the white stockings, were used, namely black and red. Black seemed to suggest death or destruction and red blood or danger. The girls, who individually appear as sophisticated young ladies, thus represent the dangers of growing up, the black being the emptiness (death) or want of worthwhileness in the child's life and the red the blood of menstruation with its challenging implications. The inviting and yet ominous figures of the girls in this setting can be seen as the unconscious guilt of sex and the unknown dangers of sex experience. The whole picture seemed to represent the repressed alarm which the child feels at the prospect of having to develop into an adult and to mix in the world of people around her.

Generally speaking, this girl's paintings were not particularly helpful to us: she was currently having painting lessons and she tended to paint set pieces. On one occasion, after we had been discussing the central theme of her inability to express feelings, she came away with a painting where red, green, blue and yellow were scrawled all over the page, painted lines of various shapes crossing each other in all directions. This was taken to represent her confused inability to handle her emotions, but could also indicate a desire to regress to infantile behaviour and to be allowed to make a mess, so in contrast was it to the exactitude of her other work. The painting thus helped in providing talking lines for the therapy.

A grammar-school boy, almost sixteen years of age, was referred to us by his headmaster because of uncontrolled behaviour. He produced paintings of two contrasting kinds. The earlier variety were of a revolting nature, mainly of grotesque blobs of mucus hanging from nostrils and other facial openings. The later ones were of an attractive

PAINTING

quality. One of these was a lake with blue hills in the distance, a green hill on the left and a grey mountain mass in shadow on the right, the red, rising sun above and colourful reflections in the water. The scene was peaceful, solitary and beautiful. The therapist's assessment of the earlier pictures was of exaggerated adolescent revolt against authority and of hatred and contempt. The other scene he saw as representing a need to escape, to ponder and to be temporarily relieved of the pressures of adolescent living.

A twelve-year-old girl was referred for shoplifting. She painted a a bridge of black stone arches with dark blue water underneath and a cloudy sky showing light under the arches. Above, the sky was dark grey with a central patch of bright red and a touch of yellow. It was a sunset scene and to the therapist it seemed ominous. Lucy agreed that it looked dangerous, but when the therapist said that the red in the sky reminded him of bleeding she said she did not see anything dangerous in bleeding. The therapist said it depended on who was bleeding and this she accepted. She said that she was bored with life.

Her next painting was of a lonely beach from which a tunnel led off. The sea was a dark grey-blue, the sky was black with streaks of grey and rain was falling. It was a dismal picture in which the tunnel represented a bolt-hole wherein to escape from reality. More dramatically than words, or even tears, could have done, it portrayed the child's disappointment with the drabness of life, her distress over the dissensions at home, her feelings of inferiority in her relationships with other children and the dawning realization that approaching adolescence – the red glow in the first picture portraying menstruation – would make new social demands.

Treatment along these lines for Lucy and later a short series of therapeutic talks with her parents achieved a measure of emotional stability.

We were asked to see a boy of eleven because he had been stealing. In the early weeks of therapy he just sat, a dead-pan expression on his face, and said nothing, unless perhaps some remark just at the end of the interview; but he painted one or two interesting pictures.

One of these was confined to the left top corner of the page, leaving the remaining five-sixths of the paper blank. A thick, black wall surrounded a patch of green grass over which reached the branch of a tree, and on this branch perched a bird. The bird was brightly coloured, black, red, yellow and blue, and he had an immensely long beak. The picture clearly illustrated the boy's situation and suggested one or two features which had not otherwise been obvious. It seemed to say: 'Here am I, shut into this little bit of the world (away up in the corner of the page), hemmed in by a wall of social restriction, but my own little patch is bright green grass. Although I am thus considered unworthy of a bigger place in the sun, I am really quite a nice bird, as witness my bright-coloured feathers and look at my beak!' Whatever other people thought of him he inwardly believed that he was a fine bird. To the therapist the beak symbolized masculine potency and also aggression against the society which had not been giving him a square deal.

Subsequent events were to prove that these two qualities, sex and aggression, were very strong forces within him. These include a violent fight which the therapist witnessed afterwards in camp and a sexual assault which led to a Court case as well as similar incidents reported by the headmaster. In the meantime the picture encouraged the therapist to talk about the boy's good feelings about himself; and an incident which took place at that time, namely a brother's wedding, provided an opportunity to raise the question of his anxieties regarding his sexual life.

A few weeks later the boy painted a ship at sea, a bright blue sea. This ship had two gun turrets each with two guns, and up in the air, above the funnel, was another gun turret, smaller and also with two guns. The therapist said, using suitable terms, that the ship represented his father, large, powerful, aggressive and sexually potent; and the smaller gun turret the boy himself with his powers represented by the penis-like guns. These latter were adrift in the air presumably in recognition of the fact that the boy had not yet established his social and sexual position, so to speak, on the ground.

An eleven-year-old boy attended the clinic because of anxiety-motivated refusal to attend school. One of his paintings was of a black and white horse, tethered to a post, while the farmer stood behind the animal beating it with a stick. On the flank of the beast were large, red scratches of blood and drops of blood fell to the ground. This obviously was a picture of the boy himself and it depicted the desperate emotional situation in which he felt himself to be.

Marcia, aged twelve, came to see us because of stealing from her mother's purse and from her brother's pocket, and because she had attacks of asthma which had persisted from the age of one year. In one of her sessions Marcia said she would like to paint and she painted a house. From discussion of this there came to light her father's readiness to yield to her and the generally good relationship she had, on the surface, both with him and with her mother. The therapist then raised the issue of the love-hate relationship, stealing being an outcome of this conflict, and of the asthma as an expression of anger. Marcia burst into tears, said that a lady up the road has asthma and angrily asserted that she loved Mum and Dad and that they loved her.

After these matters had been ventilated she painted a house on fire. The therapist interpreted this as indicative of the danger arising from these conflicting emotions as well as her fear of the asthma itself, this last being a real issue as distinct from an unconscious one, but none the less important.

A little later on Marcia elected to draw on the blackboard. She drew three figures, side by side. The centre figure was a pattern, she said. The therapist saw it as merely separating the other two figures and did not comment upon it. The second, a house, Marcia said in answer to a question, was not as good as her own. The right-hand figure showed a ship which had been blown up by the bomb, seen under the water, and two lifeboats. Marcia said that one of the lifeboats represented herself. In this sense she was at risk and was trying to be rescued from the wreck of the good family life (the ship) in which she wishes she were still integrated. The therapist said that she felt inside her also that the bomb which had done the damage was the badness in herself and that the lifeboat was the good part of herself which would save her from the damage. The house represented her home where she wanted to be happy, loving and safe. It was *her* family and it really was a very good family. The therapist noted, however, that Marcia had so far told him nothing of her feelings, had given nothing, and remained withdrawn behind the barrier which she put up. If these feelings had been expressed in the drawing nevertheless, and had been interpreted, something had perhaps been achieved.

In the session which followed Marcia talked about clothes and parties to which she had been. The therapist spoke of part of her wanting to grow up and part of her not wanting to. She said she felt awkward about meeting new people and that she was glad she had gone to the secondary school to which most of the girls in her junior school class were also going. Nail-biting and insecurity were discussed and the therapist said that he thought perhaps she would soon be able to stop coming to the clinic. Two further interviews added little more and it was agreed that she should stop, but would return after a couple of months. When this period had elapsed she came back with her mother, who said that Marcia had a much better adjustment – she was no longer aloof and she was able to be affectionate with her father as previously she had not. Marcia was friendly and she talked freely to the therapist, who noted that there seemed to have been a great improvement.

It has long been my custom to send birthday cards to children who are currently attending the clinic, and in selected cases we send a card on one or two subsequent birthdays. In passing it can be said that we have had many expressions of satisfaction on account of this and the arrangement is, therefore, one which can be recommended. It was in reply to such cards that we had several letters from Marcia, the last having been almost three and a half years from the time when she first came to us. In this letter she said she had left school and was working on a farm, helping with housework and looking after the farmer's two boys. She gave considerable detail in this pleasant letter, both about her own circumstances and about the affairs of her family, and we were left with an impression of satisfactory progress. At a still later date we received, without any initiative from us, a further letter in which Marcia said that she was married to a wonderful husband, that they had a baby and that she was greatly enjoying her present task of sending her Christmas cards and presents.

A fourteen-year-old boy, the youngest of four, was referred by a probation officer. He was an insecure child, he had no sense of responsibility, and his intelligence was at the lower limit of average. He had stolen along with others, he had run away from home alone, his parents said he was secretive, and he was known to keep pornographic books. Treatment was interrupted by irregularity of attendance, but he painted several pictures which were interesting for the naïve simplicity with which they depicted his situation.

The first was a submarine, some fish and a sea setting which he said he had seen on television. Because this was a copied picture, it was decided not to use it as a basis of therapy. Probably this was a wrong decision and the submarine and the fish may have represented members of his family and interpretive comment might have revealed stresses of the nature of which we were unaware. His next painting had a man with a crowbar who was waiting to attack a colleague, who was carrying money, derived from betting, which they were to have shared. It was a black and white effort with a faint touch of yellow and looked a bit grim. In talking to him about it, the therapist related it mainly to his hatred of society. In the next interview he painted a motor-cycle accident in which the driver was killed, and the therapist suggested that this was how, in bad phases, he felt about his own life. Bruce did not accept this interpretation, whereupon the therapist suggested that as it was his own production it must mean something from inside him. He tried to get across something of how we could at times hate ourselves, of our own guilt feelings and of how we sometimes punished and might even threaten to kill ourselves. The next painting was of a tree struck by lightning during a storm! The therapist discussed Bruce's difficulties, his feelings of rejection and his refusal to accept friendship or help. Hindsight suggests that the early features of this case might have warned of an indifferent outcome. He committed further offences and was sent to an approved school.

PAINTING

A fourteen-year-old boy whose intelligence was a little below the average, but who gave the impression of being bright, friendly and open, was referred because he had been stealing at home. It was known to our social worker that his family were considered to be the sort who would drive a hard bargain and who would not be averse from evading responsibilities. Because of his readiness to talk, treatment interviews were not as heavy going as often in such cases, but he continued to show a regrettable want of sense of duty or of concern for others. In one of his later interviews it was disappointing that he painted a picture of 'A Crook', who had just robbed a bank and who was lying on the ground in front of a policeman who held a revolver. In talking of this painting he evinced his usual, cold lack of concern and one could only hope that his evident appreciation of the power of the law would be inhibiting in view of the weakness of his own critical faculty and of the doubtful example afforded by his home environment.

Robert was nine years and three months old when he came to see us as he suffered from obsessional thinking, mainly in the form of fear of illness and of death. His I.Q. was 108 and he was elder of two brothers.

At his first interview he painted a striking picture. On the right was a boy, brightly dressed with green jacket and shoes and blue trousers, and grinning face. On the left was a much larger figure, dressed in black except for a white-and-black striped apron, brown stockings, and green necklace. She looked a fattish woman with almost leering expression. On her head was a kind of skull cap with horns. The devil symbolism was impressive. This was only the first interview, but had he not, in fact, depicted his unconscious feeling about his mother? There was some evidence for this forthcoming later when we discovered that his anxieties included a fear that his mother would poison him. With characteristic paradox he had been tearful at the beginning of the interview and was very apprehensive about leaving his mother.

In the next interview he painted a sheriff being attacked and shot by a vagabond. The sheriff in this picture had quite a similarity to the boy in the earlier one and it was easy to believe that the picture represented his unconscious anxiety, and both pictures appear as representations of oedipal fears. The vagabond is a good representation of the fantasied, avenging father. The therapist talked to him about his fear of typhoid fever, of his feeling at times that he was no good and his difficulties in facing a boy who was bullying him at school. In the next interview they talked about his own anger and his feeling of being different from other boys.

In reply to a letter sent by the therapist more than a year after

TREATMENT FOR CHILDREN

Robert first came to the clinic, Robert wrote himself, telling about his birthday and presents and saying that he was 'very well in every way'.

An adopted boy, aged twelve and a half, was referred to the clinic from a children's hospital where he had been taken as a result of anxiety-motivated refusal to attend school. Early in treatment he painted a picture depicting a parachute trooper landing in hostile territory. Two aspects of this painting were important. To begin with, it was so strikingly out of character with his timid personality that any desire he might express to take part in such activities later on in life could only be motivated, unconsciously, as a compensation for present-day weakness. There is another aspect of this picture. The parachute trooper is Simon himself, pushed out from home – i.e. the aeroplane and not in itself the most secure of possible places – into school, i.e., the hostile battleground. In discussion about this there came to light a recent incident where there had been a row at home because his dog got into the sitting-room, and about this he had become very unhappy. He had been depressed before and had made a suicidal attempt, and in this light the picture reveals his hostility directed against himself. It was difficult to believe that these adoptive parents, good though they were by outward standards, had not, in fact, been both strict and punitive throughout much of the period of Simon's life.[97]

At this stage it was impossible to get Simon back to any ordinary school, but we were able to arrange for him to attend, two or three times a week, at the remedial teaching and therapeutic play centre run by a neighbouring local authority in whose area the therapist also worked. It was, in fact, two years before he was able to return to an ordinary school, where eventually he settled satisfactorily. He left at fifteen and later we had a letter from his mother to tell us how well he was and that he had had the initiative to leave his first job because the money was poor and that he was doing well in his second.

A seventeen-year-old boy asked for help regarding indecent exposure, having been apprehended by the police. We had known him at the clinic, three years earlier, for the same reason, and his parents were warmly co-operative on both occasions, but in the previous series of interviews it had been impossible to penetrate his reserve. In the meantime he had acquired an ally in the form of a girl friend, so that on this second occasion we were not battering against the same wall of inadequacy. None the less, his degree of inhibition still appeared formidable.

The therapist discussed the patient's feeling of guilt regarding sex which prevented freedom of expression, his own inner feelings of badness in himself, and his fear of the therapist as an avenging figure who

PAINTING

is inwardly imagined as ready to destroy him if his sexual impulses are expressed. He said: 'You don't feel that I am another human like yourself. I am a kind of god-demon who would be terribly punishing if your own feelings about sex were known.' He went on to postulate how he, and mother and father for that matter, must have just the same sex feelings as the patient, the only difference of any importance being that we happened to be born some years earlier than the patient. This amount of insight had been afforded in the earlier series of interviews also. The god-demon is, of course, the oedipal, threatening father figure now deeply unconscious. The boy could accept at a conscious level that he was inhibited by shyness (fear) towards the therapist, but the aim of such interpretation is that by linking up with unconscious feeling it will neutralize a part of the super-ego pressure.

Soon afterwards the patient brought his girl friend to see the therapist and in an interview with both of them the therapist talked of their needs and of emotional pressures, in a relatively superficial manner. In the following interview a good deal was said of the patient's instinctual feelings of guilt and of the 'badness' of sex, whereby he could not exteriorize his sexual instincts with his girl friend, but could only do so secretly with strange girls (indecent exposure) who happened to be walking through the park.

To the next interview he brought a painting of a fresh country scene. This is a plan I occasionally adopt with older girls and boys, that I ask them to paint something for me at home, because this saves time, although it does not allow the therapist to observe how the patient approaches the painting. I have never adopted the measure with younger children. The present picture was of fields in green, yellow and orange, with green trees, a blue lake and grey hills under a light blue sky. The patient said that the picture represented the sort of place to which he would like to go for a holiday. On such a holiday he would walk and would fish and he would go all alone. The therapist did what he could, but without actually asking the question, to give a hint that he might enjoy taking his girl friend with him, but the patient never brought this up and even when the therapist did make the outright suggestion, the patient said he had not thought that he would want to take her. The therapist, therefore, pointed out how in the intimacy of the beautiful and lonely countryside he dare not share the joys of living and loving with her. The importance of the painting lay in the fact that it brought this out, and the therapist tried then to bring out how his irrational guilt feelings were responsible for this inhibition. Indeed, the patient said he would take her for a holiday to Blackpool, but he was somehow afraid to share with her the intimacy of being alone with nature.

The next picture was of a village street with attractive houses, a shop called 'Antiques Abbey', trees, church tower in the background and three birds. He said he might live and work in such a place. It was more social than the other. It contained his desire to withdraw from the toughness of the town, but it still left life too empty, depicting, as it did, no human activity. In these respects the painting furthered therapeutic discussion.

In reflecting afterwards the therapist considered that despite this boy's age there might well be aspects of the physical relationships of sex about which he desired information, but was too inhibited to ask. He therefore decided to cover this subject, and while talking of the detail of the sexual act he asked the patient if he had, in fact, ever experienced sexual intercourse. He said, 'yes', with his girl friend. The therapist might have wished that treatment had not brought about so precipitate a result, but it did seem that, emotionally, the patient was moving.

Blackboard drawing suits some children well and a good blackboard is a distinct asset to a clinic. Interpretation follows similar lines to that relevant to paintings, although the blackboard work has the disadvantage that it cannot be kept from one interview to another. Less inhibited children tend to go to the blackboard and it often is a spontaneous choice.

A boy of nine had been referred because of difficult behaviour involving such elements as disobedience and sulking at home and poor work at school. On the blackboard he drew an aerial war scene – planes in the air, a gun firing on the ground and bombs bursting around the planes. It was a realistic picture in which the effect of coloured chalk had been employed to some purpose, and it provided an avenue to discussion with the boy about his internal hostility, of the existence of which he realized that the drawing gave proof.

Another boy in his middle school years was referred for stealing, against a background of impaired relationships at home. His parents could be described as well intentioned but unimaginative in their handling of his problems. He drew on the blackboard a fat boy with a large head, his hair standing on end and his arms stretched out in despair. Facing him was a cannon of nineteenth-century vintage, manned by two soldiers in appropriately colourful uniforms. Fire was still issuing from the mouth of the gun and the shot was striking the fat boy on his left cheek. At the end of the interview this child asked to bring in his mother, to whom he showed with glee what he had produced. She was visibly shocked. As may be imagined, the drawing provided scope for discussion in future interviews both of the situation in which he felt himself to be wherein he was badly treated and

PAINTING

pushed around, feeling that people hated him, and also of the other side of the coin, the aggression he felt and the vengeance which in fantasy he wreaked upon his oppressors. It also provided for the social worker an opportunity to talk to his mother about the underlying emotions motivating her boy's attitudes – which she had seen on the blackboard with her own horrified eyes – and not least to explain to her that such feelings were normal human attributes, to be handled understandingly and not met by punitive attitudes or by ostracism.

CHAPTER XIII

Treatment through Relationship Formation

The value of the direct relationship between child and therapist is insufficiently stressed in current teaching of child psychiatry, yet such a relationship, involving understanding on the part of the therapist and some measure of trust on that on the child, is a *sine qua non* of good therapy. In adult psychotherapy the transference relationship is a corner-stone of treatment and in play therapy with children we sometimes have to explain to the child the existence of attitudes towards the therapist – inability to trust, aggression and others – of which he is but dimly aware. The direct relationship, factual association though it may appear to be, is actually composed of unconscious attitudes both of a postive (friendly) and of a negative (hostile) nature. For the present we are going to consider particularly children whose capacity to form good contacts with others, and to trust others, has been seriously impaired through emotional neglect. Even if their interviews are only once a week and sometimes necessarily less often than this, many of these children form a dependent relationship with the therapist and from this they are able to acquire a degree of self-reliance and, ultimately, a better capacity to mix with others than would otherwise have been the case. This can happen even when the child is so inhibited that he can confide nothing of his inner feelings to the therapist, nor is able to accept from him interpretations indicating the presence of those feelings.

We may digress here to consider *inhibition* in comparison with *introversion/extraversion* and with *ego strength*, as these concepts differ from each other, but are qualities each of which we may profitably attempt to assess as part of our diagnostic, and hence treatment, procedure. Ego strength may be described as integration, or integrity, of personality, so that the child has a strong potential capacity for adequate and fully satisfying self development. Such development may still have these qualities whether he is extraverted, so that he can achieve himself in an outgoing and euphoric manner; or is introverted, whereby his mental activities are more imaginative and gain their ends relatively more from reflection than from external action. Inhibition *per contra* represents emotional damage the result of undue super-ego pressures or of the internalization of harsh or punitive parental attitudes or of rejection, and is an inability to exteriorize oneself through fear, largely unconscious, of reprisals.

Returning to the child's inability to assimilate interpretation – because he dare not look at his own inner feelings – this will not restrict interpretative therapy in a total sense, because the therapist will still employ his own insights and with the co-operation of the social worker will leave no stone unturned in the attempt to achieve on the parents' part more understandingly generous attitudes towards their child. His own responses to his patient, mirroring his insights, are themselves beneficial.

Percy was referred to us because he had been stealing from his mother's purse, from shops and at school. He had been phoning for ambulances and he cried a great deal.

Initially Percy's mother made a good impression when she brought him to see us, but later on we saw her as intolerant, embittered towards Percy and jealously resentful of his relationships in the clinic. During one of her interviews with the social worker, when she had been running Percy down for about half an hour, the social worker suggested that perhaps she no longer liked Percy very much. At this she burst into tears. His father we regarded as aggressive and rigid.

At his first interview Percy came into the room unabashed and at once remarked on the paint, but later when painting he apologized, quite superfluously, about some of the paint having gone on the table. Such an apology is a reminder of the severe sense of guilt which these delinquent children have. He painted a boy playing in summertime and we talked of his likes at school and of the games he played. He was easily distracted and talked almost as one adult speaking to another, but at the end he begged to be allowed to take lead soldiers home, finally accepting the therapist's explanation that they belonged to the clinic.

This combination of pseudo-adult talk and a spuriously mature demeanour in a child who is disturbed in his relationships, and often accompanied by good intelligence is, in my experience, an indication of an intense need to be loved and to feel loved – a need the magnitude of which may pass unrecognized at home.

In subsequent weeks he painted the dolls' house, but did so so messily that the therapist eventually insisted on his stopping; he said he would like to do woodwork and for a time made swords using the wood, hammer and nails available, and he filled the basin with water and played at submarines. He treated the interview as a sort of playtime when the therapist was at his disposal, but without feeling that any kind of demands would be made on him and he managed successfully to reject all conversation that bore content of his difficulties.

Yet he did tell the therapist a few things. His quick eye noticed that someone had written 'fuck' on a case folder and he said this was a naughty word. When the therapist tried to explain the meaning of the word, he said 'no', that it was a naughty word. He painted an aeroplane fight and when asked if he liked fighting said that other people started on him, so he fought them. The therapist saw an opportunity to talk of good and bad feelings for Mum, but Percy would not pursue this, and *via* the construction of sand castles in the sand tray – primitive play for a boy of nearly ten, but the therapist had spoken of feelings for Mum and what Percy really needed was to be allowed to be a baby – he told the therapist that at school and in the street he was called 'cissy'. 'If I catch hold of them I'll knock their block off' – aggression expressed at last. The therapist said, 'You would like to do that?' and to this he replied, 'I would'. Percy asked if there were any birds' nests around. Where did the sand come from? What were the therapist's other patients like? He denied jealousy, but went on to ask why the doctor never put his paintings on the shelf – were they not good enough? (It is not our custom to pin up or exhibit children's paintings, but they are often left on the shelf to dry.) When the therapist gave him a birthday present he said his mother would not believe that he had come by it legitimately.

Although a certain amount of interpretive comment was made during our sessions together, interpretation was mainly one-sided in that it consisted in the therapist's understanding the meaning of Percy's more often than not negative, contribution to therapy, and what he gave to Percy was much more the quality of his own comprehending behaviour than the transmission of any insights. While transference in the Freudian sense certainly existed there was importance also in the here and now relationship.

Two more years have passed, Percy is nearing the age of twelve, he still attends the clinic fortnightly, he has a dependent relationship on the therapist, but he remains unforthcoming. That is to say that his unconscious guilt and resentment are still too dangerous to be allowed expression and his unconscious fear of punishment too inhibiting to permit exteriorization of his feelings. It may be questioned why we say that these emotions are unconscious, rather than a purposive restraint of aggression of which the child is aware. The point is that Percy does not appear to be deliberately unforthcoming, but is truly inhibited in the sense in which we have used the word. It is difficult to believe that he consciously fears the reaction of the therapist, whose attitudes he already has tested in so many ways, and a reasoned conclusion surely must be that the barriers to self-expression are internalized resistances. Percy is still occasionally stealing and we now have his parents' consent to residential schooling, which they refused when we eagerly sought it more than a year ago.

Arthian was ten when he was referred to us by his family doctor because he had stolen. He was the eldest of three and a fourth was born during the first year of his attendance at the clinic. His father had not been able to settle happily into civilian life since his discharge from the army, he suffered from bronchitis and was often aggressive in his attitudes; while his mother turned out to have a punitive streak in her bearing towards Arthian. When we wished to take him to camp she withheld her permission as a punishment and would consent only after the probation officer, who was doing the social work, had gone to much trouble to persuade her.

Arthian's treatment in the clinic was commenced on usual play therapy lines. Just after he and his mother had left the clinic from one of his early interviews she brought him back because she had discovered that he had taken with him a couple of toys from the sand tray. This was accepted with just the comment that we had to keep these toys in the clinic because they were needed for other children who came.

A year after we had first seen this boy the therapist wrote that he felt there was a recondite, affectionless quality in his character. Under these circumstances we decided that a residential school for maladjusted children was necessary, but it turned out to be impossible to gain the parents' consent. In time the magistrates placed him in the safety of local authority care.

After a year in a good children's home he was returned to his parents and the regularity of his brief, fortnightly visits to the clinic was resumed, while our camp had become his annual holiday. When he left school he ceased to attend the clinic apart from a single and somewhat stressful visit.

A case, accompanied by more direct expression of feeling, was that of a boy in his teens, rejected by his parents, who had spent nearly all his life in the care of a voluntary organization. His unconscious hostility towards those who had deserted him was projected as resentment against the house father and house mother in the children's home where he was living. During a long serious of weekly interviews the therapist acted as a sounding board for his many complaints, most of them unfounded, but freely accepted by the therapist, who recognized that, true or untrue, these grievances were genuine to the boy himself. Little attempt was made at interpretation of the projection mechanism, but the doctor listened, and at great length they discussed together his objections to the treatment to which he said he was subjected. In this way the therapist was a repository for the boy's grievances against others during a period of several months – a positive transference in which the doctor became for a time the good, accepting father figure.

Non-interpretive therapy, and especially if the therapist himself remains unclear regarding the motivation and meaning of the child's behaviour, has obvious limitations as a treatment method. It carries the risk that the therapist may be blind, while leading the blind, and the value of apparent improvement cannot be gauged, as we do not know how it came about.

Another therapeutic method which we employ, but infrequently, is the *combined interview*, at which child, therapist, one or both parents and perhaps the social worker, are present together. The instances where I have found this useful have usually been those in which an older girl or boy has felt that his parents have been persistently unfair in their demands or have discriminated unjustly in favour of a sibling. The child is apt to be diffident about making such accusations when his parents are present and the therapist may therefore have to say his piece for him, but after a time the child will usually be able to express his complaint. In a favourable case the parents will thus come to see how their son or daughter has been feeling about them and the young person may gain insight into the depth of his parents' care for him. Unless the parents have some capacity to understand and then to abrogate some of their fixed ideas and unless the child can respond with some measure of appreciative affection, such an interview is likely to be sterile and this is why the procedure cannot be used often. In selected cases it is worthy of a trial and if we can get the ice broken, with some expression of actual feeling during the interview, good will probably ensue. The aim is an improved relationship between child and parent and if it is successful it will be good treatment. It is well to allow at least an hour and a half for such an interview.

Group therapy Sometimes we have found it worth while to take children for treatment in the clinic, not alone but in a group of six or eight; and for this purpose it is desirable to collect together a group that is relatively homogeneous as regards age and intelligence. Inhibited children found opportunities to make contact with others in an environment where the intimidating pressures of school life, such as teasing by other children, were largely absent. Severely inhibited children were unable to break through from their anxieties in this respect. There was little indication that any diagnostic categories were more suitable for group therapy than were others. Perhaps if one excludes those who appear severly disturbed and regards the first three or four sessions as being a trial period one may expect thus to have a satisfactory working group.

Following Anthony[98] I have adopted the technique of commencing the session by having the children sit round a table and talk. By the end of twenty minutes one or two of them have usually begun to move away and in time I allow them to break off into play. Within wide limits they may do as they wish, and this includes permissiveness to do things which are not fully accepted in ordinary conditions, such as making a mess, attacking each other or using 'rude' words. Beyond a certain limit I curb such activity, but so long as actual harm is avoided I believe it is beneficial for children who are nervous or maladjusted to be able to express themselves with freedom and to discover that such behaviour is acceptable (at any rate within wide limits) to a responsible grown-up. For the same reason I permit a good deal of noise and hope that, during the limited amount of time when a group is in session, other persons in the building will not be unduly disturbed.

Especially during the earlier period of sitting round to talk, and also so far as is possible in the time for play which follows, the therapist will endeavour to give interpretive meaning to what is taking place. The following are a couple of examples of this. One of the boys is being aggressively untidy, throwing things about and pushing other children. I say to them: 'Billy seems to be very angry. He is making a mess so as to annoy me and is throwing things about so that he will have everything all his way. I think he feels somehow that people are bad to him, or they don't understand him, and therefore he is making us take notice of him and wanting to punish us, too, because he feels that we are bad to him. I suppose we all feel this way sometimes and it helps us to understand how Billy is feeling just now.' In another case a boy has just told a 'dirty' story or used a forbidden, usually sex-toned word, and the rest have responded with a guilty hush or snigger. I then say: 'Why is it that people say we shouldn't use this word?' I repeat the actual word myself in a manner suggesting that to me there is nothing particularly unusual about it, and I then explain its origin and what it means. It is by then probably clear that I do not regard the word or the story as being inherently evil, but I will also explain why we do not usually use such expressions in public.

The following is a note made after one group session: David whispered something sexual to Tony, which the rest of us could not hear. The doctor insisted on his returning to his seat. He refused persistently and the doctor said he must go home. As he refused the doctor put him forcibly out of the room. He returned and the doctor remarked that he must *want* to come back, that he wondered why

TREATMENT FOR CHILDREN

David wanted to come back, that he even wondered if he had been wrong in putting him out. David remained and settled down. The doctor then raised questions about why people had to whisper when talking about sex – were they afraid of it, and why was it bad? – and about why boys had a 'peter'. Following this, there was quite a bit of rude talk about 'peters', 'dirty arses' and so forth. Maurice (whose birthday it happened to be) said calmly that he thought it was dirty to touch other people's private parts. The doctor said people did not do this unless they were two people who were getting married and who might love each other so much that they wanted to do this together, and also that there were certain things people did not say. There was further rude talk and it was not possible, just as this juncture, to say anything else that would channel these feelings into a more healthy course, although indeed the expressions used were more excretory than sexual. It was now more than half-time, so the doctor said – as was his custom at this point – that they could do as they liked. They got up to play at once. A fight put David into tears and he left the room in anger. The doctor said a little to him outside about bad and good feelings and he soon returned. He attacked Kieron, and this fight the doctor broke up after a few moments. This was followed by ball play, two further fights and a barricade of furniture which was put up against George by Tony, who said George was interfering with their ball game. When the doctor said it was time to go they left peaceably.

It has been my experience that group treatment is more difficult with adolescents than with children, although a greater amount of time, a wider scale of equipment and scope for activities outside as well as within the clinic would probably be advantageous, as American workers have claimed.[99] I have never attempted to run a mixed group, that is to say a group including both sexes, of adolescents, because of the belief that such a combination of disturbed youths and girls would raise problems too difficult to handle. In an adolescent group the relevance of play will be significantly less than in a group of children, but it is not negligible and the opportunity to paint, to draw on the blackboard and to be wild together provides openings for self-expression. One group of boys for a time enjoyed throwing small rubber objects at each other.

Ginot has quoted Lebo as having concluded that 'children who reached the age of twelve do not seem to be suitable for present-day non-directive therapy'.[100] In a group of inhibited adolescents conversation may be difficult to initiate, and when one does get them to talk they want to select non-emotional subjects. One has therefore to accept that some time will be spent in talking of intellectual matters connected with school activity such as physics or mechanics, tape recorders, cars or football teams, issues which are of little real value to the children's well-being. The therapist will have to find opportunities to insert emotional concepts into the conversation; it is far from easy to get a response from members of the group and there is a risk that the therapist may become didactic. One makes an interpretation whenever an opportunity to do so is offered, one tries to avoid the session being swung too far in the direction of talk that is emotionally inert and relatively valueless – becoming able to talk on any subject in the group may be of benefit to the girl or boy who is seriously inhibited – and one aims to provide emotional counsel based on one's knowledge of the problems of members of the group.

For pre-school children Anthony has suggested that the sand tray be divided roughly into sections, one for each child and one for the therapist and that a start be made by all playing therein together. In any event a good variety of toys should be available in the playroom and the therapist must be prepared to take an active interest.

While these children form relationships with each other – superficial ones, because we are meeting only weekly and for just an hour – some of them are able to form a relationship with the doctor, and in a number of cases we have found it valuable to encourage them to continue to come to see the doctor at the clinic, usually for quite short play interviews, for weeks or even months after the particular group to which they belonged has ceased to meet. These are children whose insecurity requires this further support.

Camp. Young[101] stated many years ago that a summer camp is an integral part of a psychiatric clinic, but camping is not a usual association of most British clinics. During a recent visit to clinics in southern Africa I was told by Erasmus that children from his clinic in Pretoria camp on his farm. Our own arrangement arose fortuitously. The present writer took an active part in the running of a Boys' Brigade camp and it occurred as a natural development that boys from the clinic should be invited because they were likely to gain from the holiday. We have since added boys on probation, clients of a probation officer colleague who also takes part in the camp, and for a number of years almost one third of the boy membership of the camp has consisted of these boys. Unfortunately we have never been able to do the same for girls, because the facilities have not existed. The camp runs for eight, sometimes nine, days, as considerations of staffing and expense inevitably preclude any longer period.

Experience has shown that the camp is valuable to us in three ways. There are still a large number of children whose parents are unable to give them a summer holiday and for whom some form of organized camp is the only holiday they can get. Next is the group of boys who are poor social mixers. Some of them are, of course, too timid to come to camp at all, but for those who do come it provides a useful experience of living together, and that in an environment where they find they can survive without the presence of the sheltering parental wing. The third value we have found is that we are able to see our boys in a different and more continuous environment from that of the clinic and to discover how they operate under the various stresses and diverse circumstances which communal living provides. This experience of our children's capacities is obviously not necessary as a normal part of child guidance therapy, but there are a few boys in whose cases it can be valuable to us. It was at camp that we learned how fierce was the aggression of the eleven-year-old boy,[102] and another, who had suffered brain damage from encephalitis,[103] demonstrated in a manner which arrested one's attention how both initiative in playing and working, and drive to undertake set tasks, had been impaired by his illness. A third boy, who attended a grammar school, provided a lucid demonstration of how unintentional arrogance – the compulsion he had to display his superior knowledge and thus to argue, aggravated by the fact that he was always right – brought down on his head the combined wrath of a number of other boys, who indeed took the law into their own hands with the application of boot polish to his private parts. Yet a fourth, a rougher boy who had some delinquent qualities, displayed delightfully his kindness and affection in helping some younger boys down a rock face on the seashore. Another grammar-school boy had come to us because of his crippling lack of initiative. His headmaster had described him as a 'cow', an epithet which the educational psychologist considered unkind, but seeing the manner in which he stood in the field while others played, one could not but be impressed by its appropriateness.

The residential school for maladjusted children – the use of the term has administrative justification even if its appropriateness to the child's circumstances is not always evident – plays nowadays a sizeable and essential part in the treatment of personality problems among children. The circumstances under which we find it right to send children to these boarding schools usually fall into one or other of the three following categories. To begin with, there are those children who suffer so much rejection at home that they cannot be happy there and others where the stresses are such that an atmosphere of permanent tension and even hostility exists at home. In the great majority an underlying basis of affection remains and we find that, being separated from each other during the school term, children and parents are usually able to enjoy each other's company in the holidays, and that by the time the child eventually leaves school a happier and more stable relationship has been built up. The next set are those children who are delinquent or whose behaviour at school, and perhaps elsewhere, is incorrigibly unsatisfactory and for whom outpatient treatment in the child guidance clinic is proving to be inefficacious. The third type of child is one who suffers from school phobia or who is so inadequate that he cannot make worthwhile social adjustments, and in whose case parental capacity to provide a sense of security is so poor as to be aggravating, rather than otherwise, to the problem. These children will usually already have had child guidance treatment without benefit and the group will include a few whose presenting problem is psychosomatic.

In the words of David Bilbey,[104] there comes a time in the treatment of some of those children who are maladjusted when the workers in the child guidance clinic find it necessary to recommend placement in a residential school for maladjusted children, and it is at this point that the headache really begins. Cases are many and places too few. Unfortunately, the responsibility for placement often lies in other hands. Various methods are employed. There is the duplicated letter approach: 'The above boy has been ascertained maladjusted. Is there any possibility of a vacancy occurring in your school?' Several copies of the case papers are usually made and are sent off to a selected number of schools. In the ideal situation the psychologist gets in touch with school A for the child X because he knows the school, its head and its staff, and believes that they can help the child; or he selects school B for child Y because school B will be more suitable for handling Y's particular problems. He may be lucky and there may be a vacancy. This brings us to a very important fact about residential schools for maladjusted children. There are quite a number, all too few, in fact, but nevertheless sufficient to provide a variety of methods of treating these sick children, varying from extreme permissiveness, schools following various doctrines such as shared responsibility, schools with a pleasant family atmosphere which are imitation 'prep' schools, to schools which are just boarding schools. They all have several qualities in common. Numbers are usually small, from about twenty-five to forty; age range is usually large; they are normally located in old country houses and the policy on which they are run and the atmosphere created depend to a large extent on the personality and beliefs of the man, or preferably man and his wife, at the top.

The child who comes to the school may exhibit a variety of symptoms. He may be aggressive or withdrawn, he may wet the bed or soil, he may steal or be backward in school, he will almost certainly be

TREATMENT FOR CHILDREN

insecure, and it is more than likely that he has lost faith in grown-up people. He may have come from a very strict home or one where there is no discipline at all, or probably one where there are no moral standards. He may even have been in a remand home 'to teach him a lesson'. He is possibly on probation or he may be 'in care', meaning that he is the responsibility of the local authority.

And so he arrives at his new home and school, where at first he can relax in the atmosphere created by his new substitute Dad and Mum. He finds that there are laws for the good of everybody, but he is told about them, in passing as it were, usually by the other children. There is a whole new world for him to explore, a fire pitch on which he can have fires, trees to climb, woods in which he can play Cowboys and Indians to his heart's content, land which he can dig, and lots of aggressive work which is also constructive. There is good food and plenty of sleep and, in the background, a pleasant old horse, a knowledgeable donkey, a very understanding dog and cat, and by no means least, several understanding grown-ups who gradually prove to him that 'sickening' adults can be human after all, can love, can help, can play and can understand a child.

The child gradually becomes an integral part of the family or community and, as his confidence in the grown-ups grows, so he takes on a greater share of responsibility and begins to accept the discipline which makes the society work.

Essentially the home in which he finds himself is a place of healing and many can be healed. Some, however, have through past experience suffered so much damage to personality that they must be enabled to live with their maladjustment just as a blind man must live with his blindness. Healing takes time, but the moment comes when the child is ready once again to face up to the real world outside. In the ideal situation the social worker has been helping his family and there is a distinct possibility that he can return there, but if this is not possible then other avenues have to be explored, the hostel or more orthodox boarding schools being possibilities. The cured child is a little frightened at first, but soon adapts himself. His visits and his telephone calls and letters grow less as he finds security in his new world, while the staff left behind who have given much in love and affection feel very empty indeed, but turn to the youngster who has just been accepted – he is aggressive, wets the bed, cannot read and hates all grown-ups, but after all these were Johnny's symptoms four years ago and he has left now.

To try to lay down a set of rules for would-be workers in this field is impossible – it has been tried, but not very successfully. The people at the top should have a great fund of experience on which to draw and through this experience seem to do the right thing at the right time. They have to be sympathetic people whose own problems are solved, they must have a sense of humour, must always be ready to rebuild, often with worn-out tools. A man must be a headmaster, father, big brother, teacher, confessor all rolled into one, his wife a mother and all that being a mother entails – they must love each other. They must indeed be saints, but if ever they begin to think of themselves as such they will fail – as some already have failed.

The psychiatrist who has an assignment to the residential school can contribute in two ways. In the writer's opinion his effort should not be in treating the children but in his availability, during his visits, to discuss with members of the staff their problems and uncertainties. Often they will be reassured thereby that their handling of the difficult child is sound and they will also derive from the psychiatrist's comments or his questions, further insight into the meanings of the child's behaviour or the likely effects of their own attitudes. An occasional child is likely to require special help from the psychiatrist, in the form either of a diagnostic session or of a series of treatment interviews. In these cases I usually prefer to have the child come to my nearest clinic, rather than see him at the school.

While the child is away at school the importance of the social worker's association with his mother continues, and she will be the judge of where and of how often interviews take place and indeed of what measures are best calculated to secure good adjustment within the home for the child when he returns for the holidays and after his final departure from the residential school. Where children from our own clinics are at residential schools we try to have them along with their mothers to see us at the clinic once during the school holidays, but whether this occurs in every holiday or with lesser frequency depends partly upon the time at the psychiatrist's disposal and partly on the school's viewpoint and on the social worker's judgment.

For various reasons it sometimes happens that *approved school* is the appropriate, or indeed the only, answer, where a place in a suitable residential school for maladjusted children is not available. The vital issue in this area is that everyone in authority – the magistrates, the probation officer, child guidance staff and if possible parents also – should see the approved school as a place of necessary therapy and discipline and not as being a punitive establishment. The staffs of approved schools themselves take this viewpoint and they need, in doing so, to have the encouragement of the rest of us.

A small number of children, whose difficulties are not only a reaction to the home environment but are deeply internalized, may require shorter or longer treatment in special hospital units.

CHAPTER XIV

Some Typical Treatment Cases: the Pre-school Years and the Early Years at School

Nervous children face us with a problem of inaccessibility. We employ our techniques, we encourage play, we invite painting, we ask for dreams, we give our own interpretations of the child's anxiety and we attempt to explain his instinctive fear of ourselves which makes it impossible to confide; but when all has been done and said, some children remain silent. Obviously there is much that the child cannot say about his problem because it is not conscious to him, but there are those children who say almost nothing from one session to another and there must be much about themselves of which they are aware. An occasional boy or girl may be mute of purpose, but there must be few indeed who would come, time after time and largely of their own volition, in order to sit in silence merely as an act of revolt against the therapist. Evidently those children who will not speak are prevented from doing so by resistances that are not of their own choosing. The therapist's approach, his degree of confidence, his sympathy, his intuition and his analytical understanding must amount to a degree of skill which will vary from one therapist to another so that *one* will, as it were, possess a key which will unlock the silence of a particular child, where another therapist would fail. In practice, however, the child psychiatrist is often faced with this situation, where the reasonable degree of skill at his disposal – for without this he would be unlikely to have reached his position in the clinic – is failing to elicit from his patient any response.

One reason for this extreme reticence is guilt in relation to the problem for which the child is coming. The problem itself is due to elements such as resentment, aggression, conflict and fear, while the therapist in fantasy may represent the avenging father or mother figure of the infantile unconscious. The child will not be aware of this, but only of a sense that he cannot force himself to reveal anything of his feelings. Again, there are those children who are unaware that a problem exists except in the sense that life for them has its difficulties and family affairs their ups and downs, and because they see no problem in themselves they can hardly co-operate in attempting to do something about it. Sometimes, too, in this point of view they are not so wide of the mark, because the problem may reside chiefly in the faulty handling they receive from parents who are themselves ill equipped emotionally to meet the situations that life presents. There are some children who are aware of problems, such as the fact they do lose their tempers and become nasty or that they fail to satisfy the pundits who persist in trying to teach them at school, but as these misfortunes seem quite unavoidable they see no purpose in attempting to explore their meaning. The therapist will need to help them somehow, at first and indeed principally, through a relationship with himself. There are a number of children in whose personality structures organic factors set limits to what can be achieved; this does not justify an attitude of nihilism in therapy, but rather makes on our skill the demand that whatever can be done, and in whatever way it can be done, ought to be accomplished – examples are consultations with colleagues, daily treatment in special units, transport arrangements, or help with holidays or even finance. In one of our clinics the social worker has organized a scheme whereby, through 'Friends of the Child Guidance Clinic', considerable sums of money are raised voluntarily in order to enable a variety of projects to be undertaken, and in another there is a limited scheme for help with clothing and for assisting boys who cannot otherwise afford to come to camp. There are a few children who can be cured or satisfactorily helped by psychoanalysis alone. And there are young children in whose cases, as we have seen, better parental understanding is sufficient therapy.

In talking to children one has to be imaginative. It is almost as though one had somehow to try to get inside the child's skin, imaginatively speaking, so as almost to feel oneself in the situation in which the child is. From this standpoint, if one may be allowed to think and talk along such lines, one presents to the child verbally what the therapist sees the child's situation to be and what feelings he believes the child is entertaining. Sometimes we may ask questions, but usually as a preliminary to answering them ourselves. Sometimes we can say to a child who is dumbly offering a very bland exterior that there must be some reason why he is coming to the clinic. Possibly he will tell the therapist the reason or, failing this, he may accept it when the therapist says he believes it is because of such and such circumstances or occurrences. Another manoeuvre, to be employed sparingly, may be of use when the therapist feels he has exhausted all the resources available to him for the moment – indeed, he may feel that he is exhausted or tense and that it would be unwise to try to proceed further – is that he may say to the child: 'You don't seem to have any more that you can say to me today and I don't think that there is any more I can say. Perhaps it will be better to leave it so today and I shall look forward to seeing you next week.' In remaining chapters we shall describe the treatment of a further number of children, not so far mentioned in the text, in order to illustrate how some of these factors were handled.

I. The Pre-school Years: Children under Five
An Anxious Little Girl. Monica came to see us at the age of two years and four days with the story that she was frightened of everything outside the house, that she was specially afraid of men, but not afraid inside the house, and that she had had these symptoms for six months. She was the younger of two girls. She was said to be eating well and, since recently she had been in a bed with her sister, sleeping well. Pregnancy, confinement and puerperium were described as normal. Monica was breast fed, there were no feeding difficulties, she talked at ten months, walked at eleven months, had had no serious illnesses and had had no separations from her mother. Whenever outside the house she screamed and shouted with fright. The doctor who referred the child considered that there was an element of temper in these outbursts and he regarded the home conditions as being poor.

Although Monica's parents had been married for twelve years, they had so far been unable to get a house and the family were living with the paternal grandparents. This was an unsatisfactory arrangement, as Monica's mother did not hit it off well with her mother-in-law; she regarded the grandparents as interfering and she was on the point of tears in saying so. On the other hand, she said that she and her husband got on well together, their sex relationships were happy and the children could not wish for a better father. Cliché this last phrase may be, but as a family they appeared to be well knit. She said she did not cry often, but occasionally after a row with her mother-in-law. Having thus made an initial relationship with the family, we in the clinic felt that the most appropriate next step was to write to the medical officer of health to ask that they might have his support in obtaining a council house. As a result of this intervention five points were added to their housing priority.

At the initial interview Monica looked pale and not particularly well groomed and she did seem to tighten up anxiously whenever the (male) therapist paid any attention to her. Right at the end she was just a little more friendly. When she came again with her mother three and a half months later she looked more spruced-up, her mother was obviously happier and she said that Monica was less afraid of strangers. When the social worker visited a year after we had first seen them, she was greeted by grandmother, who told her that the family now had their own council house, that Monica had largely got over her nervousness, though she still was shy, and that things were much better for all of them, the mother-grandparent relationship especially being more friendly than it had been. More than six years after the initial visit Monica's mother, in a letter, said that Monica was very well and added that she, the mother, appreciated all we had done for them. Indeed, we had done little, but we probably had done the right things and had done them at the opportune time.

This baby's emotional upset must have had some meaning. There were appreciable elements of stress at home and a degree of resultant tension between mother and father was likely. One could hazard a guess that overheard parental intercourse or bed-time argument had produced a fear of men, as threatening, and thus a conflict between her spontaneous love of her father and this fear. Factors, broadly of this nature, probably were operating; but if the reader is reluctant to go as far as this with us, we can still see that the stressful home situation caused a feeling of insecurity and that this amounted to panic when she had to leave her home and enter the (even more frightening) outside world. We recognize with our older patients that an inability to face the outside world of school or of adult society has stemmed from the insecurity of inner relationships at home. Cannot a baby be agoraphobic for similar reasons?

The Demanding Child of an Anxious Mother. A little boy, Marcus, was almost four years and two months old when he came to us, referred by the medical officer in charge of infant welfare because of temper tantrums, disobedience, screaming, quarrelsome demandingness towards his sister and bossiness with other children. Marcus was the younger of two children, and although by superficial standards the home was a happy one, there were appreciable stresses. Maternal grandmother had died when Marcus was a few months old and mother had suffered after this from neurosis which lasted for a year and was treated by the family doctor. A maternal uncle was currently an in-patient in a mental hospital. Father was a somewhat rigid man, a worker in the distributing trade. He was not in full agreement that Marcus should come to the clinic; he could not understand why mother was 'making all the fuss', and he said that he blamed her and that she was 'a bundle of nerves'. The origin of the problem we regarded as being: 'Mother's anxieties and insecurity and father's want of insight and his inability to provide her with support, with consequent lack of a stable home background'.

Mother twice had threatened abortion at the three to four month period of her pregnancy with Marcus, but otherwise pregnancy, birth and the post-natal phase were satisfactory and Marcus was breast fed. Developmental milestones were normal and toilet training did not seem to have been excessive, but as an infant he cried much if left alone and as he grew older he became difficult to manage insisting on having his own way in everything. On the occasions when he played with other children he must be the boss. If his mother took him out shopping it was clear that 'they were paying scores against each other with Marcus usually bringing off the bigger success'. If his mother had friends in to tea he would upset the party by saying that his mother must not speak to her friends and by repeating this frequently. We decided to give Marcus a series of treatment interviews in the clinic and that the social worker's support for his mother would be important.

Marcus seemed a warm child, not seriously maladjusted, and he took easily to playing in the clinic. In his first treatment interview he played happily in the sand tray. He put *all* the pieces in the sand and said he did not know what they were doing – an indication of impairment of conceptual capacity in a child whose I.Q. was 114 – but he chatted freely about his Christmas presents and said he could play football. He then played ball with the therapist for a little time. When he rejoined his mother at the end of the interview *she* became excited about his gloves and shouted, 'Marcus, Marcus', to which Marcus paid no attention. Taking this along with the history, it was not difficult to imagine causes of the anxiety which must underlie the impairment of his conceptual capacity which we have just noted.

In the next interview he wanted to paint. The painting was very much a smudge and he did know what it was meant to be, but he did agree that he sometimes was cross with his sister and with his mother, that he then felt they were naughty, but he could not say in what manner. He seemed to be afraid that if she were cross she might leave him and when the therapist put it this way he agreed. In the next interview he was more detached and did not know what he wanted to do. The therapist suggested this and that at which he might play, but little emerged. The following interview was missed and the one after that was similar to the last, except that he wanted to go back to his mother after twenty-five minutes and this the therapist accepted. Generally one would try to use the remaining time, or part of it, to discuss or discover reasons why the child is so anxious to return to his mother, but the child may be too anxious or too inhibited, and in any case the issue must be decided on the circumstances of the moment.

Father came with Marcus on the next occasion and asked if the therapist could help to get him a place in school next term, when he would still be some way under five years of age. The therapist had, in fact, spoken already about this to the principal school medical officer, and this new little piece of pressure from father was further indication of the parents' desire to obtain this external solution to what was far more a problem of mother's anxiety than of the child's, largely resultant, behaviour disorder. Marcus was happier in this interview and the therapist made a note to the effect that he believed that he would improve slowly and that he considered it unnecessary to go on with treatment for much longer.

Fordham once said that he tended to divide his children's cases into those which could be dealt with quite quickly and a remainder who would require prolonged treatment. In my own experience it has become apparent, from the point of view of sheer economy in child guidance treatment, that the great majority of problems presented to us are to be dealt with by a régime of treatment which is both purposeful and brief.

The relationship which the therapist had with Marcus at this time was still a pretty tenuous one. He drew three pictures – a head, a girl's head chopped off, and a man. Asked what he would do with the girl's head, he said he would bring it home for lunch. Asked if he would like to eat the girl's head he said, 'No'. Asked what would happen to the girl when she had her head chopped off, he said that blood would run out. The therapist considered that Marcus had, in fantasy, murdered his sister in this drawing. He felt, however, that unless he had been meaning to proceed more deeply in treatment – which seemed unnecessary and was probably inappropriate – it would be a mistake to arouse deep anxieties and thereby probably to bring about even stronger repression, by making any such interpretation. It was probably of some value that anxiety could be released by Marcus producing such a drawing and by the therapist's receiving it as one that could be accepted and talked about naturally in the way they did talk about it.

The next interview was the last and the therapist asked if Marcus remembered his drawings of the previous week. Marcus said he had forgotten them and the matter was left there. He then painted a tortoise going to the water – an apt simile of his own slow progress towards the happiness of that self-realization which sets us free to live our lives in a worthwhile manner.

Treatment had covered a period of four months from the date when we first met Marcus, or two and a half months from the time when treatment interviews actually began. Fifteen months after we first saw him our social worker saw his mother, who expressed herself as being well satisfied with developments. He was, of course, by then at school. More than eight years from our original meeting with Marcus our social worker got into touch with his mother once more. She herself sounded very anxious and said that she had been having treatment from her doctor. She said that Marcus was still highly strung, but had adjusted well to the secondary school. Only once since his discharge from the clinic had they had difficulty with him. On that occasion he was for three weeks very unwilling to go to school, but his parents found out that he was being bullied and they were able to deal with the matter. Considering the background of parental emotional limitation, this was perhaps not too bad a result.

A Child with a Specific Fear. Thelma came to see us at the age of four years and two months, having been referred by her family doctor. He phoned to say that she was terrified of spiders and that he would be writing us, although his letter did not turn up. Her treatment consisted in no more than to discuss with her mother the circumstances in which the child found herself, in order that partial understanding of what was happening in the child's mind would enable the parents better to handle her difficulties.

Thelma was the elder of two children of artisan-class parents in their middle twenties, the younger child being a boy of sixteen months. The problem as stated by her mother was: 'I cannot seem to get through to her unless I shout and then she gets upset.' She had started the previous year to scream the moment she saw a fly and would scream if a fly flew past her. She would get on the floor, kick and shout hysterically 'Kill it, kill it.' She said that all insects were bumble bees. (There was no record of her having been stung by an insect.) She was afraid to go out or to go to the lavatory, all from her fear of flies. She slept well, but took a long time to get to sleep, and a few weeks before coming to us she had been waking up in the night and screaming about flies. Her mother said that she herself had as a child been afraid of spiders and would scream, and that Thelma's father did not like spiders, one having dropped on his face when he was a baby. She also said that if Thelma were outside sitting on a blanket and if flies came she would cuddle down behind the baby as though wanting him to protect her.

Thelma was born at home, the second stage of labour had lasted at least three hours and terminated in a low forceps delivery with extensive tearing. She was breast fed for two weeks and then weaned to artificial feeding, despite her mother's having a good supply of milk, on the doctor's advice. She was not a happy baby and cried a great deal, especially if put outside in the small garden of the caravan which was then the family home. She talked quickly, saying 'Mum' at six months, other monosyllables by a year and sentences soon afterwards. At eleven months she had started to walk, but she fell out of bed just before one year and did not walk again till thirteen months. Toilet training was started at ten months and was not easy, but she was almost dry by two years and completely dry by night at two and three-quarter years. As a baby she would not be cuddled, but by the time she came to us she would sit on a parental lap. Sometimes she would say to her father in the evening :'Do you love me? I have been thinking of you all day'. An abscess on her chin, due to the fall from bed at nearly twelve months, had to be opened in the hospital outpatients department, and two months before she came to us she had fallen in terror of a fly and as a result had developed an abscess on her back. Her I.Q. came out at 100+.

She enjoyed looking at pictures in books and drawing with wax pencils – she drew circles with legs sticking out, which were spiders. It was not easy to keep her interested. She played reasonably well with other children and was friendly with the little boy who lived next door.

Her parents' marriage was described as a happy relationship. Both parents were affectionate towards the children and both had minor traits of insecurity. A small matter which arose months afterwards caused us to wonder if mother's sense of responsibility for Thelma was just what it had seemed. A 'follow-up' interview was arranged. As they did not turn up and did not send any letter, we wrote to ask mother if she would like an alternative appointment. To this there was no reply and when later our social worker went to visit she found no one in on three separate occasions. On the third occasion she saw a neighbour who told her that the house in question was occupied by Mrs X, a name in no way resembling that of the patient's family. Eventually she discovered that Thelma's mother was Mrs X's daughter and after a great deal of research she eventually found her at an entirely different address. This was a not unintelligent family and we find that such straws in the wind can be an indication of the manner in which parents evaluate their children's affairs.

Return to our initial interviews with mother and child. When I first met Thelma she had had her session with our psychologist, but she would neither come with me nor even look at me. I accepted this and told her that it would perhaps then be better if I just had a talk with her Mum. This brief meeting had taught me that the little girl's anxieties extended beyond insects to people. Her mother was friendly and seemed capable of understanding my explanation of her child's difficulties. I first of all discussed the position that if she were able to understand the child's problem in a general way and that if she then attempted to support and encourage her, this would probably be the best therapy. I outlined my view that Thelma had been one of those children who just had more difficulty than most in coping with the inevitable frustrations of childhood, beginning with those of breast feeding. She had therefore felt rejected as a baby, had inevitably responded by feelings of aggression, had found it difficult to give love, refusing to some extent, because of her own bad feelings, the love that was given her. I went on to explain how, a little later in her babyhood development, she would have become jealous against her mother in relation to her father. When I mentioned this, her mother said that Thelma had always become upset if she sat on her husband's knee. I explained how this jealousy would cause the child to feel further aggression and how she would in turn feel bad or guilty because of this aggression. It appeared to me, I said, that at the age of two plus she was in this sort of emotional turmoil when the baby was born. This event must have thrown her into a state of consternation and hatred and desire to get rid of the baby. Her mother then told me that Thelma had said that Mummy and Daddy should not have had this other baby. From her destructive feelings about the baby there must have arisen further fear of punishment and of rejection. As these emotions receded into the repressed unconscious, somehow the menace they contained became attached to insects, hence her irrational terror of these creatures. No wonder reasoning had no power against this fear which could be allayed only if she could become more confident of the efficacy of her parents' love and of her ability to love them. Thelma's mother appeared able to grasp my outline description of these matters and it was decided that she should come again after three weeks. It would not be necessary to bring the child on that occasion, as direct treatment for her was not considered necessary.

At the next interview her mother said that all had been well until the day before, when Thelma had been terrified by a bumble bee; and she also mentioned one or two other things that she had not told us of in her initial interviews with the social worker and myself. She said that if Thelma were reproved, such as for throwing stones which might hurt people, she 'behaves as if she had been shouted at' and sulks terribly, burying her head in a pillow. Later she would apologize. Obviously such reproof, however mild, serves only to stir up wells of tremendous guilt arising from the deeper issues which we have discussed, and if her mother and father could understand all this they might be able to handle such incidents as the stone-throwing in a more imaginative and constructive manner, the long-term results of which would be better than would any kind of scolding. 'Do you really need to throw stones, because they might hurt one of these boys?' will probably be met by the reply: 'Yes, I do, because I want to hurt them'; but this sort of going-along-with attitude on a parent's part is actually of more use than saying: 'You mustn't do that', at any rate to a child who is as guilt-ridden as Thelma was.

Her mother also said that Thelma still wanted to be rid of the baby, yet when someone in a restaurant took him to show to someone else, Thelma screamed and said they would not bring him back. At times she was very loving towards the baby. The incident in the restaurant reflects her own deep anxieties on account of her death wishes against the baby, whereby if the baby died or were stolen away it would be her fault – this is, of course, unconscious, but it results in the fact that if the baby is in any actual danger, then she is acutely afraid.

When our social worker eventually found Thelma's mother later on it was almost nine months since we had first met them. She said she had had no further trouble with Thelma, there was no more trouble with insects and she was now able to take more affectionate interest in her little brother.

Nardil and librium have been recommended as adjuvants to psychotherapy for phobias in older children or adolescents.

II. The Early School Years
Children at this time may be as yet in the genital phase of emotional development, when feelings of love, sex or aggression are freely expressed and when interpretive comment along these lines are still acceptable. Even if this phase is passing from them, they remain in close relationships with parents and siblings, and if the repression and resultant inhibition which come with latency have not set in it should be possible to discuss some of these relationships in crude form. In practice this is often far more difficult than our theory would suggest, because relationships have been strained, guilt fantasies repressed and emotions of rejection are too painful to be contemplated.

Anxiety Symptoms in a Neglected Child. Stanley first came to the clinic two days before his sixth birthday. He had been referred by a school medical officer who had been impressed by his mother's, all too genuine, tale of woe. Stanley had a facial tic and other obsessional movements, he had nightmares, he suffered from headaches, occasionally he wet his bed, he was a poor mixer and his mother described him as being 'not a lovable child' who was aggressive with other children. The educational psychologist had noted that during half an hour while he witnessed Stanley's behaviour in school there were no tics. There was one elder brother and it was evident that both parents tended to reject Stanley if he were 'difficult'.

Stanley's mother was friendly, co-operative and at times vivacious but in other moods she was depressed and apathetic. She was sensitive to Stanley's behaviour. His father was an apparently cheerful, friendly man, but was subject to mood swings and inclined to be impatient with Stanley, although obviously fond of him. He had run into a good deal of trouble on account of motoring offences, for the last of which he had just been in prison and Stanley had missed him badly while he was away. By trade he was a lorry driver and it was his stupidity, rather than any badness, that got him into these difficulties. Elsewhere in the notes he is described as a ditch cleaner, so that he must have changed his job. He had been married previously and had two grown-up daughters who were not with the present family. It was difficult accurately to assess this family, but our feeling was that they could be described as indifferently happy, with Stanley tending to take the blame if things were wrong. At school Stanley was said to be well adjusted, not to have the tic, but to be slow in learning. His I.Q. was 93.

Our assessment of Stanley was of an insecure child who had suffered a measure of rejection and whose great need was to feel wanted and loved and to be encouraged in his own activities. Our psychologist gave him an apperception test and this indicated to her: Fear of loss of his place to someone else, aggression towards his mother and a desire to side with his father. His dog, which had been killed, was said to have been the one creature by whom Stanley felt he was loved. In the year before we first met him he had been having phenobarbitone, which his family doctor had prescribed for the reason that it was only with this aid that his mother could control him.

He was a rosy-cheeked, sturdy but odd-looking, undersized boy, a shade clumsy in his movements, and he came into the playroom willingly. Asked about school, he said he did not like it. Asked what he did and did not like at school, he said he liked painting but not arithmetic and did not like his teachers. In reply to a question about the other children he said in a mumbled sort of way that they were 'all right'. He played purposefully with the toys, but his interest was poorly sustained. At the second interview the therapist asked him what he would like to do. Stanley walked around with his hands in his pockets, grunted and finally said he would like to draw on the blackboard. He drew a house. The therapist asked if it was his home and he said it was not. The therapist then asked him about his home. Stanley said they lived in a bus, that he slept with Roger and that his mother and father slept together. Then he stood around with his hands once more in his pockets. (It came to our knowledge at this time that his mother had been telling other children that Stanley was to go into an institution. We had already been aware that she wanted to have him sent away to a residential school.)

In the next two interviews he munched crisps and ate sweets from a packet held in his hand, he drew a ship with crayons, he played with the wooden blocks, he wandered around and picked up a pistol and he painted a field. The therapist asked if he would like to talk about what we could see in the field and Stanley said, 'No.' The next interview was missed and in the one after that he said that his mother did not want him to paint for fear of harming his new suit. (Some clinics provide aprons for painting. I have not found this necessary, but on occasion have tied a towel round the child to keep her clothes clean.) It was quite difficult to get any rapport with him and the therapist asked if he would like to play snakes and ladders. Stanley declined this, saying he did not know it. During the interview he said very little spontaneously, but it was possible two or three times to get a faint smile. He said a sore mouth had kept him at home last week, but it was now better. The therapist decided at this time that he must try to have a talk with father.

When Stanley was firing shots from guns in the playroom the therapist asked him if he sometimes felt so angry that he would like to shoot somebody. Stanley nodded and smiled. Later the therapist asked something about school and Stanley said school was 'all right'. The therapist said: 'The first time you came here you told me you didn't like school.' Stanley said: 'I like it now.' He continued to be distractible and played with guns, skittles, cutting out paper with scissors, painting, hammering pegs, sailing boats in the playroom sink and washing articles that he had painted.

In his ninth interview Stanley said that his father had fallen off a lorry and broken his leg. This was accepted factually and an opportunity seems to have been missed to explore Stanley's feelings about his father, regarding which he had so far revealed very little. The injury, however, turned out to be a less serious one and at the next interview father came with Stanley and had a talk with the social worker, seeing also the psychiatrist briefly at the end. He appeared as cheerful and friendly, strikingly like Stanley in appearance and manner, and he seemed to think that he was now understanding Stanley better than he used to do. He mentioned that while he was away in prison Stanley had refused food and pined for him for three days. The social worker felt he was endeavouring to take a constructive interest in Stanley. We shall anticipate here. Stanley's father was not a particularly intelligent man and roughly two years from the time of which we have just been speaking he had, within a few months of each other, two further accidents, in the first of these having had a smash on his motor cycle and fractured his scapula, while the second had occurred while he was driving a caterpillar tractor, and on this occasion he injured his foot so badly that the local general hospital was unequal to cope with it and he was transferred to a regional special hospital. About the same time mother had a gynaecological operation as a result of which she felt 'infinitely better'.

This accident proneness on father's part is, of course, germane to the whole family problem of which Stanley's difficulties were a major part, but it was only now that another interesting episode came to our knowledge. Stanley's mother told the social worker that when he was between a year and eighteen months old he had a childish ailment for which he was having large white tablets and penicillin injections. The night before the last injection he was 'dreadful – he bounced up and down on his pillow all night. He did not cry, but he did not relax at all. His father and I will never forget it – we both cried before morning'. Another stressful incident had occurred about eleven months after the interview with the therapist last mentioned when father came with him. On this occasion the family had just moved out of the bus in which, as Stanley mentioned in an earlier interview, they had been living, into a bungalow, and Stanley had a change of school. He had been at the new school for a month when 'nerves' developed again. He complained of pains in his head, shook his head violently and his whole body twitched. His mother said that he cried all night on that occasion. We regard these incidents as being evidence of emotional instability rather than as indicating any genuinely organic disturbance.

Several months later again we had from another reliable informant a statement that Stanley's mother habitually neglected her two boys, going out to work, leaving them to prepare meals and sometimes failing to get food for them to prepare. This informant also told the social worker that mother had herself been in trouble with the police for stealing – irrelevant, perhaps, but yet another straw in the wind. She also said that in a month when Stanley stayed with maternal grandmother his behaviour and appetite were very good, these both being points on which his mother had made complaint.

Return to the ninth interview, some two and a half months after Stanley first came to see the therapist – his original visit to the clinic had been four or five months earlier than this. At this interview the therapist said that he might soon be able to stop coming. Stanley readily agreed and it was arranged that there should be one more visit. The previous week, in fact, his mother had said that there was considerable improvement, and the therapist considered that whatever had been achieved was probably the optimum for the time being. In the tenth interview the therapist noted how insistent he was on doing everything for himself, such as putting water into the paint pots, which was something the therapist normally did. He also spent a bit of time drinking from the baby's feeding bottle in the clinic – often a sign of desire to return to babyhood care. He also remarked that it squirted like a water pistol – a urination fantasy.

It was a year later that the family moved and we heard of the return of Stanley's nervousness. After we had considered the situation a note was made to the effect that we felt mother was ready to off-load Stanley's problems on anyone else. We considered taking him in a group we were running in the clinic, but the transport situation presented a difficulty. Five months later the family doctor asked us to see him again. He would not leave his mother alone and was following her around, but she at least said she could now bring him again to the clinic, using whatever transport was available. The therapist wondered whether the task of getting Stanley to talk about his feelings of being rejected would take a disproportionate number of interviews and whether it might not be better to be content with an attempt to patch up matters in a few sessions. Stanley was eight years of age now and it would be quite difficult to obtain better exteriorization of feelings than had been possible with the younger child of eighteen months ago.

Subsequent interviews, of which there were ten in all, were not dissimilar from those of the previous series. He played freely with a wide variety of toys, water was prominent in his play, he sucked at the feeding bottle, but he made only weak contact with the therapist. In one of his sessions he painted a chapel. The therapist asked about this and Stanley said none of the family went to church, though he used to go. He said he would rather not go to school either, but would prefer to go to work with his father. When the therapist asked about trouble at home he said that he sometimes did get into trouble and he agreed that his mother did not understand what he felt, but he could express no detail. The therapist made a note of how typical Stanley was of the inhibited, 'working-class' boy who cannot exteriorize feelings. In the ninth interview of this series the therapist asked about school and Stanley denied the existence of any difficulty other than that he did not like school. Only when the therapist told him of complaints from his teacher, which mother had relayed to the social worker, did he admit that there was any trouble. The therapist accepted Stanley's version of what had happened and said that he thought the teacher had not understood his feelings and that it must make Stanley unhappy when he was not understood. Stanley agreed. He got hold of the baby's bottle and sucked away at this. The therapist asked him if he thought it would be nice to be a baby again and to be fed and loved and looked after. Stanley said it would. In the next interview he seemed to feel at home and to be content, but he was reluctant to talk and chose to play by himself, although displaying an awareness of the therapist's presence in the room.

But for the transport problem to which we have referred already, we should probably have taken Stanley in a group this time, rather than in individual interviews. This it now became possible to do and he attended group sessions for the next few months. Almost seven years then elapsed during which time we were not again called upon to help. Our social worker then called on a visit of enquiry in connection with our survey of earlier cases. Stanley was several months beyond his fifteenth birthday and was on the point of leaving school. He hoped to join his father, who was by this time working in forestry. His mother said he was much improved, although he still had some symptoms such as blinking and a facial twitch, and there were occasions when he shouted out in his sleep and was excessively active.

Looking back on Stanley's treatment after the passage of years, it is clear that help was needed. The more necessary part of treatment, however, was probably the help we could give to his mother in order to assist her in accepting him as he was and, to some extent, in handling her own problems of resentment and of frustration. It is at least arguable that more purposeful concentration on this aspect of the case might have justified the therapist in dealing with Stanley himself in a briefer series of interviews, and might thus have saved time with much the same result as was actually achieved.

This last point raises an issue that we have not so far dealt with in these pages. Occasionally it happens that the mother requires this kind of help, but specific therapy for the child seems unnecessary, yet the mother is reluctant to accept that she needs 'sorting out'. Under these circumstances it may well be right that the child should be taken for a short series of treatment sessions in order that the mother may receive from the social worker what she needs, without loss of face.

Phobic Anxiety in a Young Boy. The case of Tom is interesting as showing how a fixed fear was treated in interviews which involved one or two sand scenes which were pictorial representations of internal anxieties, along with a preference to relate to the therapist in a 'safe' or factual manner. His age was six years and nine months when he came to us, his I.Q. 132; he was the elder of two children and the complaint was that since the age of two and a half he had had a fear of steep slopes and was also afraid of P.T. at school or of anything adventurous. Once or twice he had written backwards. Sometimes he saw things, such as the clock, the wrong way round. He was afraid of almost any height, of going up, of going down or of being in the middle of the slope, and he did not like going on a swing.

The pregnancy, delivery and puerperium had been normal and there was nothing unusual about Tom's early life except that he was a little late in walking and talking. His parents were naturally affectionate and seemed patient and understanding. Mother had a limb deformity and an additional disadvantage was the crowded and unsatisfactory condition of their home in a condemned property as a result of which mother had often to curb Tom's play activities. At the age of two and a half Tom went into hospital to have an operation for a pain in the groin the medical nature of which mother never discovered. He was in hospital for eight days, was very upset at having to leave his mother when he went in and became disturbed when she visited him, but was quiet when she was not there. It was soon after he came home that his mother began to notice his fear of coming downstairs, of slopes generally and of large floor spaces. This appears to be a case where the separation anxieties – and whatever unconscious fears from the pre-genital or oedipal emotional complexes were reinforcing these anxieties – have become displaced to this fear of slopes. It is not a fear of slopes as such, therefore, but the fear of slopes is representative of much wider and deeper anxiety. The factor which decided that slopes should be the object of the fear may have been the circumstance that when he was seperated from his mother, on going into hospital, he was carried upstairs by an ambulance man and was very distressed by this separation. His mother noticed afterwards that on some hills he was very distressed, but was usually all right if he was against the right side wall. He was not a demanding child, but was loving to his mother and father and was very sensitive, for example if he heard of anyone being hurt. The support from the wall may be symbolic of that from mother.

Tom was a good-looking, friendly child, who came willingly into the playroom and decided to play with the sand. He expressed his anxiety at once by gasping that his baby sister 'drives me mad' – he had just had to look after her while the therapist had been talking to his mother. The therapist thought it would probably be adequate to see him a few times. As it turned out there were twenty interviews in all.

In the next interview he was inhibited and evasive, had difficulty in finding anything to do and eventually chose to play snakes and ladders. This he enjoyed and then he tried the xylophone. At the next session he made an aerodrome in the sand and then a farm. In this there was nothing obviously emotional. The therapist asked if he had been on a farm and Tom said he had only passed one. He painted a boat and said he had once had a sail, but that they were not having a holiday this summer. He did not, of course, say these things spontaneously, but only when the therapist asked him. In the session after this we talked about his birthday and presents and his party. He said he liked other children and was fond of his sister, regarding whom he had earlier expressed the frustration. He made a farm in the sand.

At the following interview he asked to play snakes and ladders and after this he made a sand scene with horses and cattle. These attacked some 'Indians', who were vanquished by them, whereupon cowboys attacked the 'Indians' and some of the cowboys were killed by the animals. Next a big fire brought many trees down, one fell on an 'Indian', there were a few other incidents and finally rain put a stop to the fire. Later a number of 'Indians' dug for themselves a hollow in the ground and shot from there. The animals seemed always to come off well. From the notes it was possible to make at the time the therapist seems to have said very little about this scene in the sand. It obviously was representative of warring emotions of a 'good' and a 'bad' kind within the boy and also perhaps to some extent of feelings of what he would like to do to certain figures in his life outside. This representation of these things in play could be beneficially cathartic in itself, but it would be of advantage if this effect were reinforced by a remark or two from the therapist along these lines.

The five following interviews were similar to several of the previous ones, with a strong leaning towards playing snakes and ladders with the therapist, and in one interview as many as three games were played. In one of the interviews he said he was going to make a scene in the sand of people climbing hills! He added that he was no longer afraid of slopes unless they were muddy and slippery. Following this group of interviews there was one with another sand scene of 'cowboy and Indian' type with much action – stampedes, clashes, 'Indians' climbing trees or hiding behind them, trees brought down by 'Indians', animals running about, an animal lassoed and animals killed. This scene was discussed with him only on a matter-of-fact basis. About this time his mother told the social worker that he was better as regards heights, but was apt to get into a rage if, for example, she wanted him to wear a 'mac' in bad weather, that be became upset and cried about such things and that he was afraid of going out to play in the dark. In the next interview the therapist worked round to this matter of fear of the dark, leading up to it by a remark that we were now into December. Tom said that he was not afraid of the dark, but added that he used to be. We talked about being angry and he said that his little sister spat, kicked and bit and that his mother allowed him to smack her for this. (This was later confirmed by his mother.)

In the next interview there was a sand scene of a great fire with destruction and death, but afterwards he resuscitated all. From this it appeared to the therapist that Tom was able to feel that dangers and anxieties could be overcome or dissolved and he referred to the possibility that harm could be put right and that when things were dangerous and frightening we could grow up not to feel any more afraid of them. Several subsequent sessions followed a similar pattern and at the eighteenth interview we felt that we had done about as much as was necessary and Tom agreed with the therapist that two more times would be adequate. In the nineteenth interview his school and Sunday school were mentioned. He admitted to having been afraid in school, but he said not now and seemed happy in saying so. In the final session he wanted to play ludo with the therapist and he won this game. He said: 'I like coming here', but was willing to accept that he did not need to come further. His mother expressed satisfaction with his progress.

Although not occurring until some time afterwards, the zenith of Tom's progress in relation to his fear of heights was when he went to Paris and ascended to the top of the Eiffel Tower. Our last news of him was eight and a half years from our original meeting, by which time his mother said that he was a big, strapping lad who loved football and was generally a very normal, easy-going sort of boy. At grammar school he was generally in the first eight in his class.

CHAPTER XV

The Middle School Years

One might say that in the early school years we have to provide opportunities, in play and in our commentary, for the child to express his thoughts or feelings, whereas in the middle school years which are the latency period we have somehow to interpret the child's situation and to feed it back to him in a manner and in doses which he can accept.

An Anxiety Neurosis which had become Internalized
Arthur had been referred to the psychiatrist in the adult clinic, who prescribed librium as a temporary measure and passed him on to us. He was nearly ten years of age, the elder of two brothers, and his I.Q. was 133. He suffered from widespread anxiety, he had difficulty in sleeping, he felt that people did not like him, he worried about trivialities, he was very self-critical and became most upset if he could not complete some task he had set himself, he had said he was daft because of something he had not been able to do, he worried about illness, he had severe outbursts of rage in which he could be very nasty to his mother and he used to 'take it out of' his little brother. He was described as a difficult boy who had slept poorly from a few days old until he was five and had again been sleeping badly in the last few weeks before he came to see us. If his mother left him when he was a baby he screamed until he vomited. Weaning had been difficult and he was finicky about food. Toilet training was easy, as he 'seemed to take over on his own'. His school reports were good, although he worried about lessons but when he first went to school he had been sick and was given phenobarbitone.

There was evidence that mother had been unduly anxious when Arthur was a baby; she told us that she had had too little milk and that he had had to be bottle fed at two weeks and she cried as she said this. It is difficult to estimate the probable effects of mother's anxiety. Parental inadequacies and conflicting attitudes had played a part, but we suspected that Arthur had aslo suffered from an element of constitutional emotional weakness. His father was described as so good that he would never leave him to cry, although in recent years he had been much less patient. Arthur's little brother was a more confident child and mother seemed to feel that she had been able to give him a better start. Mother and father appeared to be happy together and their relationships with each other, and with their friends, to be satisfactory. Nevertheless, mother continued to be anxious, over housework for instance, and father to be tired and irritable after a hard day's work as manager of a department making electrical equipment.

Arthur was friendly when he came to the therapist and willing to discuss his symptoms. When painting was suggested he mentioned that he had been first, equal, at school but added that it was not quite honest to say so! In the next two or three interviews Arthur painted an Alpine scene, a Welsh seaside scene, a bird and many butterflies. It turned out that he collected butterflies; he had some knowledge of country life and some time had to be spent on talking of these things. He also told of his keenness to become a sixer in the Cubs. In talking of butterfly physiology it came to light that micturition and defecation in his home terminology were both 'going to the toilet'. When the therapist raised the issue of his symptoms Arthur referred to boys who were unfriendly to him and especially to one, Terry. He said that Dad had a lot of headaches and 'is ever so strict with us when he comes home', especially if he had had a difficult day at work and was in a bad mood, but it was his mother who told us that he was again sleeping badly and wanting to come into his parents' bedroom. One or two of his paintings allowed the therapist to refer to Arthur's own relationship needs, but it was difficult to get anywhere below the surface of his feelings. When the therapist raised the issue of aggression Arthur was ready to talk of boys who annoyed him at school and his father's unfairness in sending him early to bed: he spoke with some pressure of anxiety, clasping his hands, but avoided mention of his own feelings. The therapist was still in doubt as to the nature of the nuclear problem, but in the next three paragraphs we shall see this emerge as his feeling of inferiority, his jealousy and his sense of being rejected.

If a boy paints butterflies and wants to talk about butterflies because he is interested and has a collection at home, the therapist will have to assume some interest in the subject, as he would otherwise be rejecting of what the child is offering to him. Yet this sort of preoccupation can provide more of an escape from than an avenue into discussion of emotional difficulties. The therapist therefore limited the time devoted to this subject and he asked about issues previously mentioned. Arthur said he had offered a bolder front to the boy who bullied him at school and that this had given the boy a bit of a shock. Experience shows that this kind of statement is often wishful thinking and represents what the child is trying to resolve to do, rather than what he actually has done. Even so, it may be a step in the right direction and the therapist may either accept it, or if he is genuinely disbelieving he may say he wonders if perhaps this was what the child was trying to do, but that perhaps he has not yet quite managed to do it. He asked about daydreams and Arthur said that he imagined himself as scoring goals in important football matches. He added that he hoped to get into the school team next year and that he might be the eighth best player! A few days later he dreamt that he was a Queen's Scout and that he had won the Duke of Edinburgh's Award.

After about four months the therapist had the impression that there was a measure of improvement, but the social worker's information from mother was to the effect that much was unchanged and that Arthurs's jealousy of his brother, his nasty temper and his anxieties about going to bed were still prominent. He had many fears and worries and was talking about wars and death. She formed the opinion that mother was spending much time in nagging Arthur, that she was intolerant of his awkward behaviour, unduly complaining of her husband's attitude and unable to relax herself.

Arthur could at this time be seen as an intelligent boy who had a great drive to succeed, as in Scouts and football, but who countered this by a strong sense of unworthiness and self-criticism, as seen in the instances where he deprecated his achievements. He was demanding of love from his parents, but had a constant feeling of rejection, shown by his hatred of his mother, his rages and his attacks on others. As a guide line to future therapy it was apparent that Arthur needed help in grasping that his mother and father really cared for and believed in him, and we had to recognize that there was a small amount of circumstantial evidence which, to Arthur at any rate, would make it appear that this was not altogether the case. It could be a beginning if Arthur felt that the therapist understood him and appreciated his real value and his aspirations, and whereas insight was not easy to achieve through direct interpretation, its eventual achievement might be helped considerably by a strong relationship between child and therapist. The social worker had also a valuable task to perform in that if mother could be more relaxed the benefit of this would accrue to Arthur. About this time the therapist found an opportunity to discuss reproduction and Arthur asked if excessive masturbation would prevent a boy from having a baby later by using up all the semen.

There was further talk about the boy who bullied Arthur and this was also discussed between the social worker and Arthur's mother, because the latter had been sufficiently concerned about it to pay a

MIDDLE SCHOOL YEARS

visit to the headmaster. This appeared to have a good effect. There was an instance when Arthur was going to paint a picture in the clinic when he wanted a pencil, but did not ask for one. The therapist commented on this and Arthur said he was shy and he said how hesitant his voice was when speaking to 'strangers'. It was good that he was able to share this with the therapist. He went on to complete his picture, which was of nineteenth-century naval warfare, shells hitting the water. The therapist contrasted his inner aggressiveness as shown in the painting with the shyness to which Arthur had just referred.

A few weeks after this mother told the social worker that Arthur had said to her that the therapist had been talking about the birth of a baby and that he was disgusted. This was especially interesting in view of what Arthur had said about masturbation. It shows how inevitable this guilt is in the child of a conventional British family and the meaning is that Arthur had to confess the sin of this talk on sex and his interest in it, the confession being necessary to absolve him from the guilt. Some time afterwards the therapist brought this up and said how his reaction had been an indication of how he felt bad inside about something which was both natural and lovely.

In subsequent interviews there were further instances of his strong tendency to self-criticism and his mother referred to how enraged with himself he sometimes became. Both from Arthur and from his mother we heard a good deal more of the strong hostility that sometimes arose between Arthur and his father and Arthur said how his father became angry and red in the face, threw him down on the chair, which hurt his back, and how his father sometimes said he was sorry and tried to make up for it. He was not quite so forthcoming about the strength of his own anger. The therapist explained how father had perhaps been unable to express his anger during his own boyhood and how he (the therapist) considered that it often was better to be able to express our angry feelings when we were young.

By this time the therapist was feeling that Arthur had turned the corner on the road to mental health, although he noted that he still gnawed at his nails and was still insecure. It was decided to stop treatment after the next interview.

Five months later he came back with his mother, who reported substantial improvement. Arthur painted a scene with horses and immediately said his red colouring of the sky was not good. The therapist said that if ever he were short of money he might sell some of the pictures which Arthur had painted for him! After a further seven months he and mother again returned, mother saying that Arthur was consistently better, although he still displayed much aggression against his little brother, that he still lacked confidence and had been afraid that he had typhoid fever. On balance, however, things seemed to be going pretty well and no further interviews seemed necessary. In all it was nineteen months since he had first come to the clinic. Eight months later the therapist had a letter from Arthur in which he said he had passed the Eleven plus and had been attending a grammar school for some months. 'I find it very interesting with the new subjects. I hope you are well.' This sounded satisfactory. Nevertheless anxieties returned the following spring regarding school games which were played after school hours and it was necessary to allow Arthur to return to the clinic for a time.

Imaginative Talking as a Technique in Therapy
Norman was thirteen and a half when he came to see us, this being a re-referral by himself and his parents, as he had attended the clinic some years earlier, although from the records it appeared that little had been attempted in the way of treatment. The symptoms were, as they had been previously, stammer and bed-wetting, but the stammer was much improved by the time of this, later visit. Norman had never been dry and the wetting now concerned him much, particularly as it restricted his ability to go on tours organized by his school. He was the younger of two children. His mother said that at the age of five he had been frightened and cowed by the children next door. As a baby he had been affectionate and cuddly and his mother described him as being now, at the age of thirteen, quiet and placid, yet argumentative, continually active and always up in arms about real or imagined injustices at school. The family doctor considered that Norman wet his bed when he was anxious or depressed and he had prescribed medicine for this without much success. His I.Q. had been assessed at 129 and he attended a grammar school. He was not without friends.

Norman's mother had been depressed during the pregnancy and she had always been mollycoddling and protective and had not helped Norman to learn to do things for himself. It was not until after he was twelve that she allowed him to ride a bicycle, as she was terrified of road traffic. His father was assistant manager of an industrial department; he appeared to us to be a generous man, but we wondered if he, too, had not, by accident rather than design, also dominated Norman. Their relationships appeared to be good, they both enjoyed sport and attended football matches together. There was some evidence of rebellion on Norman's part against maternal restrictiveness, as when he had said: 'Oh, Mum, don't be so fussy. I'm growing up now, I'm not a baby any more.' But his father said he showed little aggression and that if he became angry he cried. It was clear that Norman's deeper emotions were under much repression and the therapist considered that this overcontrolled boy was likely to present quite a problem in treatment and that much would depend upon whether or not he could be got to exteriorize feeling.

In the first interview Norman was diffident, but he had come for help of his own free will and he was willing to talk. He said he was happy at school, was especially fond of athletics and games, but enjoyed some of the academic subjects also. He had always wet his bed, he stated, but could be dry for two to three weeks on end. The second interview was heavy going and when the therapist brought up the subject of girls Norman denied any interest in girls and said he cared only for football, cricket and the like. He even said he wished he was at football at that particular moment instead of in the clinic; he stood up to look out of the window at boys who were playing in the clinic garden – a distraction with which we are faced in this particular clinic by the remedial teaching aspects of its programme – he tapped his fingers on the arms of the chair and he gave a low whistle. After the therapist had said, for the second time, that he did not think Norman was taking matters seriously, tears came into Norman's eyes. He said he wanted to go on a trip abroad with a party from school and that boys would tease him if he wet at night. He wept openly. The therapist said that boys who behaved in that way were not mature themselves and that the mature boy, the sort who might have a girl friend, would be more sympathetic. Norman was at this stage unable to make any kind of positive contribution and the therapist decided that he must try to force issues a little. He therefore talked about shyness, how universal a quality it was and how shy boys and girls were of each other up to the age of twelve. He spoke of how shy a boy was of a girl seeing his penis and how shy a girl would be of a boy seeing between her legs, but that when we got some way into our teens these things altered and boys and girls began to feel differently about each other. Norman was silent, but by this attitude he evidently accepted what the therapist said.

In the next interview the therapist encouraged Norman to paint and he painted a scene of animals in the primeval forest. Norman was unable to be forthcoming about this scene except to say that these primitive times and animals of long ago interested him, but the picture gave the therapist an opportunity to speak imaginatively. He said the picture was an illustration of the wild feelings inside him, the wide freedom of the forest, the dangers presented by the wild animals, the natural instinct of these animals to fight, to love and to mate, to forage for their food, to emit their excretions when and where they felt like and sometimes to inspire fear in each other. He tried to elucidate how all these functions were natural, and could not therefore be inherently wrong, how each had its own emotional value and how, deep down, Norman himself had all these same crude desires. He elaborated on the origin of fear, first in the crude tooth and claw of the jungle and afterwards in ourselves in relation to the things we wanted to do as little children, things of which our parents were disapproving, and of which as infants we had therefore become afraid, imagining reprisals or punishment. In this he tried to get across to Norman some understanding of our inner feelings of guilt.

Two interviews were missed, one of them because of sports trials at school and the other for some other reason. When it happens that a child who is attending the clinic has some competing interest, such as a special occasion at school, a party or some other occasion which has emotional importance for the child, I consider that he should be encouraged to go to that function, if he wishes to, even if it means missing an attendance at the clinic. I believe we should always pay respectful regard to what things have significant meaning in the child's social life and his fantasy life. It is nice to be told if an interview is going to be missed and such occasions sometimes are opportunities for strengthening our relationship with a child. It can be useful in the following session to ally oneself with the child through asking about the occasion and how successful it was.

In the next interview the therapist invited another painting and Norman depicted a cave dweller hunting deer. He said he would not like to live that kind of rough life, but would prefer the present, more comfortable existence and that to his mind the painting was just a picture without reference to his feelings. The therapist, however, insisted that he thought a part of Norman did want to break away from convention, from regulation and from safety into a more free and more challenging existence. Norman agreed that there probably was something in this.

At the next session Norman was silent and the therapist stressed how afraid he was to utter a sound and by pressing the absurdity of this state of affairs he was able to get Norman to volunteer the information that he had, along with others in the team won the football medal. He went on to say that the exams were due to start on Friday and that he liked exams, but did not not say so because no one else liked them, not even one boy who was very good at school work. The therapist suggested that Norman must feel proud of winning the medal and Norman agreed. The therapist tried to get it across that it was healthy to have a feeling of pride on such occasions. Concerning the exams, he said that perhaps it was sound policy to keep quiet about unpopular emotions that one might have, especially if there was no great principle involved.

The going was difficult and the therapist decided that what Norman could not say he should try to say himself, thus talking imaginatively for him. He therefore asked Norman about his feelings for girls and Norman replied that he had no time for girls, as they spent so much time going around with boys to the pictures and other places. The therapist remarked that to say that one had not *time* to be interested in girls sounded like saying that one had not time to eat or time to go to bed and that Norman's statement thus seemed unreal to him. He then referred to masturbation, telling Norman that this word meant the habit that a great many boys had of playing with one's own sexual organ, to make it feel nice, which was something that boys were doing really instead of having a girl. This he said because he believed that it must strike a note of feeling from the experience of a boy of Norman's age and capacities and in order thus to bring into the open the existence of a live interest in sex. Norman said that he knew nothing about this and the therapist said he did not see how Norman could help having feelings – he surely must sometimes feel that he would like to kiss a girl, to touch her body or to see her body. Norman replied: 'Of course I do, all boys do.' The therapist said that perhaps he was shy of girls. Norman replied forcibly: 'No I'm not shy . . . when we go out I walk with girls.' The therapist said that Norman had reacted strongly to his remark about being shy and that when a person responded with such force it often meant that the thing he was denying was really the truth, which by insisting that it was not true he was trying to hide from himself, let alone from others; and that perhaps he was indeed very shy of making a loving approach to a girl, deep down within himself, and that he greatly wished he were not so shy. The therapist felt that such admission as Norman had made of his sexual thoughts must be worth something, but that it was inappropriate to try to press this matter further for the present.

The therapist was anxious further to explore or to exteriorize Norman's fantasies of badness in himself, unworthiness, frustrated omnipotence and anger. It was not so much that there was direct evidence of these emotions, but that they must be important in an ambitious boy of Norman's considerable ability yet restricted expression. In this connection the stammer was relevant. No good opportunity to discuss these issues arose and they were not, in fact, brought out during the treatment as fully as the therapist might have wished. A more extensive investigation of the boy's personality would not only have been time consuming, but sometimes it is as well not to try to bring to the surface personality traits that may in themselves be providing useful social drives and are not directly responsible for present symptoms.

A couple of weeks appear to have been missed after this and at the following session Norman was able to tell the therapist of considerable successes both in athletics and in academic subjects and he was justly pleased with himself. He seemed a good deal happier than he had been and he said, spontaneously, that he had not had a wet bed for six weeks. There was some discussion about his plans for a future year, although several years remained before he would be sitting the G.C.E. examination. The therapist noted that it might be possible to stop fairly soon.

Two weeks later it was possible to say that neither stammer nor bed-wetting had troubled him for a considerable time. The therapist raised one or two issues which he felt to be still outstanding and it was decided that treatment could be discontinued subject to one more visit to the clinic a couple of months hence. When Norman again came after that period he was happy and was acquitting himself satisfactorily.

The Paramount Importance of Interpersonal and Family Relationships in the Middle School Years

Gussie's case is interesting because of how little we were able to do in a difficult family situation, except that we did manage to keep in touch and were rewarded by news of promising progress a number of years afterwards. Gussie was eleven years and three months old when he was referred to us by the dermatologist with the complaint of periodic, severe, urticarial oedema of face and neck. He had complained of feeling dirty before the rash started and was very conscious of his appearance when it was present. He slept poorly, had a fear of dying and was described as quick-tempered and sensitive. His I.Q. was 94, performance score only 87 and verbal 101, which suggested poverty of adaptation to affairs, but he had a number of hobbies and was a moderately good mixer. He was the fourth child in a family of seven, he had been artificially fed from birth, his mother had pot trained him from birth and her story was that the urticaria had followed a fall from a tree at the age of eight.

There was a tale of considerable friction at home, especially when Gussie was younger. His mother was much on the defensive, self-righteous and voluble in defending her brood where any argument arose, and it seemed to us that this was a home where the mother cared for the material requirements of the family, but had little understanding of their emotional needs. Gussie's father was said to have been difficult to live with, but to have learned the art of playing with the children. Our social worker described the marriage as emotionally dead. The maternal grandmother said that 'The children would be much better if my daughter had more patience. She is always shouting and bawling them down.' We could not exclude a constitutional element in the origin of this urticaria and the oedema which accompanied it, but we considered that Gussie had been submerged in the middle of this family and dominated by his mother's personality and by her greater incentive to keep up appearances rather than to provide her children with unselfish love, while father's poor capacity for family leadership was a relevant factor.

Gussie was a good-looking, well-built, friendly boy who came willingly to his first interview with the therapist. He was moderately free in discussing his situation, but he minimized a series of school difficulties of which his mother had made great complaint and he played down the severity of his symptoms although his mother said that he had had a severe attack only a few days before. The therapist considered that the mother's complaints were largely founded on fact, but that the sense of injury she felt over a wide area of experience was an exaggerated one, and that she was suffering from much complex inferiority and resultant sense of injury. We decided to take Gussie for treatment, but there was an inevitable delay of a few months.

In his first treatment interview he was diffident, but with a little encouragement he got round to painting a farm tractor. No more could be done than attempt to establish contact on the basis of everyday affairs. In the next interview the therapist attempted to talk around the subjects of his known interests, symptoms and fears. He denied both the feeling of dirt and the fear of death. In view of what happened shortly afterwards one might question the wisdom of even alluding to these matters at so early a stage. They had been freely mentioned by his mother as among her reasons for bringing him to the clinic, and yet the inner sense of unworthiness attaching to the bodily deformity and the sense of rejection and guilt involved in the death fear – in origin a punishment fear arising from oedipus and sibling jealousies – were matters of which he was too self-conscious to allow of their being ventilated with somone whom he had not yet learned to trust. At all events Gussie refused to come to his next session and, indeed, the therapist never saw him again. Six weeks later the social worker called at his home, where she saw him looking very well and where she learned that there had been no recurrence of the rash. We were therefore content to leave it at this.

Almost six years later the social worker made a further call. With some difficulty she found a maternal aunt who told her that the family had moved to another part of the country five years previously, but it so happened that Gussie had been with this aunt for the past ten weeks. Gussie had left school at the age of fifteen and had taken a job in a garage where he was earning £11 a week, but he was so unhappy with his family that he had run away from them ten weeks previously and was now living with his aunt and working as a farm labourer. He was much happier and he seemed to be having no trouble. The aunt made the comment that her sister had made a mess of the whole family and had been quite incapable of giving them what they needed; she had been inconsistent, lacked mother love and was always trying to keep up appearances. She substantiated these charges with many stories and the social worker believed her, as her account of the matter was similar to what the maternal grandmother had said years earlier.

The Child who has Problems, but who cannot Co-operate in Therapy
Among the most challenging situations we meet in child guidance are those involving children who appear to have great need of treatment, but whose co-operation in therapy is so poor as to raise doubt as to the worthwhileness of any attempt to help in this way. In some of these cases an attempt to press therapy would be traumatic to the child and the best treatment will be to temporize; and at the same time to give to the parents the help they need in order to enable them to adopt the not very easy attitude of standing by almost passively while their child seems to be at risk. In others, a relationship with the therapist, even if tenuous, may be better than none and some interpretive comment will be of value even if not fully accepted. We try to avoid giving interpretations for which the child is quite unready or which he is bound to reject.[105]

The case of Rose is interesting in this way and also from the angle of diagnosis which was a matter of some uncertainty. She was eleven years and nine months when she came to us, referred by the surgeon to whom she had been sent on account of abdominal pain. We discovered that she had attended another child guidance clinic for a short time several years earlier and the geography was such that, although that clinic was in the area proper to her local authority, ours was more accessible from her home and our colleagues at the other clinic were quite happy that we should take her over. It is highly desirable that those responsible for administration area-wise should try to meet the reasonable convenience of patients in matters of this kind. The referral on that occasion had been for a phase of school phobia, but when she was brought to see us the story was that she had actually broken into the school and had thrown things around in the dressing-room. We were also told that, in addition to the abdominal pain regarding which the surgeon had been consulted, Rose was not a good mixer, she had been subject to screaming attacks and was still histrionic in her behaviour; she had outbreaks of temper in which she threw on the floor whatever was in her hand, and although she was attending school she was very sensitive to physical education and showers. Four years previous to her coming to us she had had alopecia and nightmares in which she screamed: 'Leave me alone: I don't want to do it.' Later in the same year the social worker from the other clinic had found her to be an unwanted child who resisted school, sulked and was inhibited; and her mother had at that time described herself as 'a bag of nerves as a result of what has been happening'. Although we ourselves never discovered this degree of rejection of Rose on her parents' part, if our colleague's appreciation of the situation was an accurate one it would provide a much simpler explanation of the psychopathology than any that came to light in our own clinic. Other comments from the very good earlier social history were that mother was one who blew hot and cold so that Rose was overprotected at one point and rejected at another, while father appeared to be not really involved in the family but to put on a strict act. Rose's intelligence quotient was assessed at 91 and her headmistress said that she appeared to be completely withdrawn, quite untruthful, and a girl with whom they could make no real contact. One earlier incident was interesting. Rose had been taunted by other children at school for being 'a cry baby' and had rushed home for the carving knife with which she had set out to attack them. The therapist assessed her as a child who felt rejected and who felt unloved over a wide area of her relationship. As regards a treatment programme, he felt that the aim should be to try to get across to the child the feeling that he was genuinely interested and affectionate. On that basis he hoped it would be possible to give her the support of a relationship and in time to discuss her problems with her.

In the initial interview which she had with the psychiatrist Rose's mother said that Rose got on pretty well with her father and that he spoiled her. If we define the spoilt child as one who has been denied an attitude of loving and unselfish discipline from his parents but has been pampered by concessions mostly of a material kind, it is easy to see how the spoilt child may become the difficult older girl or boy. Her mother also said that Rose got on fairly well with her, that she 'played her up' somewhat and swore at her sometimes, and that she, in return, had tried everything except hitting Rose. In her initial interview Rose looked glum and as though she did not know whether to co-operate or not. She painted a seaside scene and said she had been to the coast on holiday. The therapist was left with the feeling that he had still to make friends with her. Despite the warnings contained in the notes from the other child guidance clinic he felt that he had, at this stage, little understanding of the inner nature of her problem or of its origins. In order to leave as much time as possible for talking during the next interview he asked Rose to paint something for him at home and to bring it with her.

She brought with her a painting of a sea scene. On the land side there was sandy shore and further along a black rock, while out at sea was a rock with a lighthouse built upon it and in between were a number of little ships. (It was only when they met mother after the interview that the therapist discovered that part of the painting had been done by Rose's brother and to some extent this may have affected its validity as a representation of Rose's feelings.) The therapist interpreted the mainland as being mother, protecting and caring but also dangerous (the black cliff), the lighthouse as being father, dangerous in its rocky aspect but welcoming and safe as the light itself, while one of the ships close in by the shore could be herself, afraid of the big sea and perhaps of some of the other ships which might chase her. The rock and the lighthouse might, the therapist said, also be him, because she wanted him to help and he could show the way to happiness perhaps, yet he was also dangerous and threatening.

In the next three interviews Rose did not show much interest in painting or any other activity and the therapist had to make the going by a combination of asking questions and by making suggestions or interpretations, either by way of comment or by way of answering the questions he had asked. In this way a number of things were either revealed or agreed between them, mainly as follow. Girls at school tried to borrow things, Rose declined and arguments resulted. With boys she had no association, feeling that they were a rather dangerous kind of animal. Her elder brother, who was crippled and lived at home – between him and Rose were a sister and another brother both married and living away – sometimes got annoyed and upset her so that she cried, but at other times he played with her, and she wished that her father could understand her feelings better than he did. Rose agreed that in some ways she did not feel as good as her contemporaries and the therapist talked of her resultant resentment and hating. She agreed that her attack on the school was a punishment to the school, as she said for those parts of the school programme which she disliked. This raised the showers and undressing question – it was not the undressing but the temperature of the water that she disliked – and when the therapist asked about her periods she said they had actually started in the previous week. The doctor talked about shyness, boys and girls seeing each others' bodies, and Rose said she did not know about babies and birth. The therapist said they must talk more of this and afterwards he wrote to her mother to say that he planned to do this unless she felt that the matter had already been sufficiently covered in talks at home. A few days later the police phoned the therapist to tell him that Rose had unlawfully entered a house and stolen money four weeks previously. The inspector agreed to let her off with a caution on this occasion.

The next four interviews can be taken together. The therapist mentioned the phone call from the police and Rose said that a friend who was with her was more at fault than she and the therapist accepted this as perhaps being the case. In the case of a child who so much needed acceptance and love it seemed safer to do so than to point out how her complicity amounted to her being almost equally responsible along with her friend, although the therapist's relationship with her was such that he could have adopted the latter course as being more strengthening to character. Rose painted a man sweeping fallen leaves – the date was April 4th – and this led the therapist to ask if life sometimes seemed not worth living, to which Rose gave an affirmative answer. Exploring this, the therapist asked something about her father and she said that she wanted him to do things that he did not do, such as playing cards with her, but that he said he was too busy. The therapist was reminded of the note by the social worker years ago to the effect that father was insufficiently involved. Rose brought a pattern she had painted at home of squiggles, zigzags, crosses and suchlike. She said she did not like squiggles and preferred zigzags. She said she was enjoying her Easter holidays, mostly in the house doing housework which she liked, and she added that she sometimes 'played up', such as turning the wireless on full and running upstairs when she was alone with her grandmother. The significance of this became clear only afterwards in the doctor's interview with Rose's father, and a year later when her mother told us that Rose had been a good deal happier as a result of her grandmother having left them. The therapist talked about sex, as he had said he some day would, including references both to menstruation and to masturbation. Rose appeared to assimilate these comments despite the existence of a barrier to any mutral discussion. On another occasion she brought some drawings which she said she had copied, as she had been unable to produce anything herself. The doctor said how she was thus unable to tell him anything of herself.

The doctor had an interview with Rose's father at this time. He was a passive but friendly man who did not produce much spontaneous comment, but he said that Rose liked to boss him. He regarded her mother as stricter than himself; he said she had thrashed Rose betimes, though seldom of late. Grandmother had been so dominating towards Rose that they had had to put a curb on her activities in this connection. He also mentioned that the elder brother, the crippled one, had given up his work with an instrument-making firm some years ago and would do no more, and that he was apt to complain about Rose.

In the following few sessions it was difficult to make headway. The doctor found that Rose seemed, though passively, to enjoy sitting on his knee and he encouraged this. Rose was absolutely unspontaneous; she could find nothing to do in the clinic and she hardly said a word for several sessions on end. The doctor spoke of what he imagined to be her difficulties at home; he referred to jealousy which she faintly admitted, he talked of his need to find out more about her, he suggested that in some ways she felt different from other girls and he said that perhaps there was something that she knew was at the core of her problem but did not want to reveal. Rose said she had told no one and did not want to tell the therapist. The therapist said that she was probably afraid of what he would think of her if she told him and that he, of course, understood that sometimes a girl felt she had to solve her own problems by herself. It was interesting, at the end of one of these sessions when every opportunity had been given to Rose to say something of herself and when she had maintained total silence, to be told by her mother that Rose had refused to go to school. This was mentioned virtually as they were going out through the door and the doctor does not seem to have taken the chance this would offer him at the next interview to say how guilty she must feel about her fear of going to school and how uncomfortable it must make her to be different from other children in this way, and thus to show that he understood.

The doctor wondered, though in the absence of any actual evidence, if a sexual assault at some time could have a bearing on the problem now. He raised with Rose every possible issue about which she might be anxious and when she painted a picture and could say not a word about it he went so far as to give her some of his own associations to what he saw in it – death, a hospital, a snake and parts of the human body – and indicated what possible meanings for her such things might have.

Seeking for hunches in his own mind, the therapist came round to saying to Rose that he thought she was feeling a tremendous need to be loved and to be wanted – by father, mother, the therapist himself, and her friends – and that she yet felt somehow that she was not allowed to have this love and that she had to make herself do without it. He said he wondered if perhaps she was worried because someone had done something naughty with her like touching parts of her body and he said that even if such things did happen he did not feel they were as bad as people often said they were, especially because they were usually loving, as well as naughty, acts. She denied that anything like this was the case, though only after a moment or two, by a slow, half-hearted shake of the head. Asked if she felt ashamed or bad in herself and if she knew something of why, she admitted that this was so.

Rose brought some paintings she had made, mere patterns they were, but she had used beautiful colours, and the doctor said that there were beautiful things in her, but that they were difficult to get out. She said she was 'fed up', that she would rather not go to school, but would like to stay in bed all the time. From this it came out that she felt her mother and father gave her better love and care if she were in bed, so that what she felt was they did not love her enough when she was well. The therapist could not get her to say any more on this aspect of her feelings and in a couple of further sessions little happened, although in one of these she seemed to be biting, picking and gnawing at her nails more than ever. The doctor referred to this and said how she was longing for love, how she felt inside like the little baby who was sucking milk from her mother's breast but felt she could not get either milk or enough loving, so in sucking and biting at her fingers she was having to suck and tear it out of herself.

To the following session Rose brought pictures she had drawn of space men. She said she thought they were funny, but the doctor said he wondered if they were not dangerous and powerful, and that she felt she wanted to have this power and freedom. She did not accept this, but the doctor said he thought it must be there inside her. He also remarked on what in the drawing looked to him like male genital organs, using words that she would understand. The doctor asked if she could tell him anything of what she felt or even what she had been doing. Rose mentioned a row with a girl from next door, slightly older than herself, the girl having said that Rose put her dirt on the pavement and that she (the other girl) did not like sweeping it up. The doctor spoke of how we could have good feelings for our own dirt, of how a baby valued the excreta which it had produced and how we could feel good about our own waste products. The next two interviews did not produce much and the doctor took an opportunity to speak of sexual things once more and about perhaps wanting a boy friend to love her and to do loving things to her. The only response to this was finger-biting and picking with a nail, which probably meant that Rose had some awareness of the correctness of what the doctor was saying, but that she could not yet face up to the realities of this situation.

These words hardly give a picture of the actual situation. Rose, good-looking, friendly and apparently warm-hearted, willing to come to the clinic and to co-operate in non-verbal ways, was one of the most passive children the therapist had had in treatment, and apart from an occasional nod or shake of the head, infrequently a word or two and rarely a sentence – apart from these she was inhibited and mute. Of unconscious hostility and desire for love there was plenty, but in a conscious sense she was an accepting but reserved child. The therapist knew of occasional outbursts of anger which occurred at home and these and her stealing, as well as her very detachment, were the most obvious signs of inner aggression. We knew also of her paucity of real friends and there was the incident of the carving knife of which mention has been made already. Even her paintings gave little indication of the anger lurking underneath the surface, and it is a criticism of the therapy thus far that although anger was sometimes mentioned there had been an insufficiently purposive policy on the therapist's part to bring it out.

In the next interview the therapist was again trying to elicit from Rose what was the nature of the conscious problem of which she was unhappy, and he worked round to what he said were his own feelings about Rose's essential goodness. This led her to say that her anxieties involved a girl two years older, with whom Rose had been friendly, and that this girl had done something that was hurtful or damaging to someone else. It was not a case of stealing or lying but of something hurtful. She would reveal no detail, and in what way she was implicated or whether the older girl was merely symbolic of guilty elements in herself could not be discovered. In the next session she painted a picture of three girls, playing at tig in the park, of whom she said she was not one. She said that this had nothing to do with the problem we had been seeking to find out about and the therapist wondered how far the immediate problem was that she had no real friends and that other girls did not mix well with her.

Shortly after this Rose said that she no longer wished to come to the clinic, because she was now missing biology, which she liked, in order to come, whereas she previously had been missing English, which she did not like. She did not say this outright – Rose said virtually nothing outright in the whole time she was coming – but the therapist was able to drag the information from her and it amounted to that statement. This frustrating, yet constantly challenging therapeutic effort had now lasted through eight months and now it was crowned with this irritating, rejecting comment.

The first question to be pondered when a child makes a remark of this kind is whether it represents what the child actually feels or whether it is a rationalization and if there are other, more complex reasons why the child wishes to stop. If she had merely asked to alter her time of coming we could have accepted what she said at its face value, but unless we have valid reasons for believing that the girl or boy has a conscientious interest in not missing some lesson, we can be certain that the child who wishes to stop coming to the clinic is motivated by factors that mean more to him than a subject of the school curriculum. It may be just that he is not happy in the treatment situation and if that is so it usually will be better to stop the sessions and adopt a different way of helping the child and the family to handle the problem. I believe one should be hesitant about attempting to press for a continuation of interview therapy, but if in the exceptional case the doctor decides that this is the proper thing to do, then he surely must alter its nature in some way which will make the child feel happier about coming. There may, of course, be some other reason, such as that children at school are asking awkward questions about where he is going to every Wednesday afternoon, and if there are reasons of this kind they require appropriate adjustment. If it seems too unflattering to the therapist that the child should wish to discard him for a biology lesson, one has immediately to recognize that what is important is not the success of this form of treatment but whatever is going to be of the greatest over-all gain to the child. It may be that this form of therapy in the hands of the therapist is not his most useful contribution to the welfare of this child. If such is the case, he obviously must alter the programme.

The present instance was not the first in which the doctor had wondered if perhaps the time had come to discontinue regular treatment, but when he had asked her about it previously Rose had indicated to him, by the aforementioned gestures of nodding or shaking her head, that she wanted to keep on coming. This time, however, she did seem more ready to stop, and as the therapist had considerable doubts about the worthwhileness of continuing the treatment much longer, he decided that this was the right moment at which to make the break. He also tried at this time to discover a little more about current friendships and was rewarded with a story about how she and her friends climbed trees after school, and on Sundays, in the churchyard. It was impossible to avoid seeing the irony of a situation where this girl, whose capacities for loving, social empathy and enjoyment of living were so deeply buried beneath her own sense of resentment, guilt and unworthiness, was finding her best social recreation to be in simian (rather than more highly socialized, human) activities among the graves of her ancestors! She said she did not go out much with her parents and it came to light that she was dissatisfied because she had to be in at 7.30 in the evening while other children's parents allowed them to be out till 8.30. The therapist saw this not as a reality situation – how far it was or was not true, in fact, seemed to him to be relatively unimportant – but as an expression of dissatisfaction with her parents and of her own intrinsic need to rebel and to feel independent, and that it actually was an exteriorization of her unconscious sense of being rejected. What he said was that she was annoyed with her parents because they would not let her do what she wanted and because she felt they did not understand how she felt, and that she had to punish him also by always looking sad and keeping her mouth shut during the sessions. She told him that she could laugh and talk in the churchyard and at home. The therapist indeed felt that by this time she had gained a degree, minimal perhaps, nevertheless real, of self-confidence and a sense of being accepted and wanted, which would be enough to allow her to progress without further regular visits to the clinic. It thus was easy for them to agree that she should stop coming.

Rose came back to see the doctor by arrangement three months and six months later and it was on the second of these occasions that her mother remarked on the improvement since grandmother had left. Reviewing the case, the doctor considered that the nuclear problem had been that of a child who had a severe sense of being unwanted and that from this all her troubles stemmed. Furthermore, a scrutiny of the social history reveals that beneath the surface of this family's apparently well-ordered life there were subtle stresses of some magnitude and parental attitudes involving emotional neglect which were probably sufficient to account for much of the girl's personality disturbance.

The therapist had believed that at this stage Rose and her family could be left to carry on under their own steam, but the following year he had letters from her headmistress and her doctor to the effect that Rose was suffering from headaches, feeling tired and sometimes going to sleep for most of the day and was refusing again to do P.T. in school. It was apparent that Rose was afraid of other girls at school, she was resentful and she felt inferior. She would divulge nothing and the therapist suspected that he might have been missing an underlying depressive neurosis. He therefore prescribed parstelin, 1 mg., daily. During the following months there was a slight improvement and the dose was reduced after a time to 1 mg. on only five days per week. The evidence for a diagnosis of depression remained inconclusive.

We did have a letter from Rose three months after she left school. In this she said that she had started work and that she liked working much better than she had liked school.

A Psychosomatic Symptom in Relation to Family Stress
Hiccough is not a commonly encountered symptom in child guidance practice and the following case is of interest both from the nature of the symptom and on account of one or two other features. It illustrates how the symptom may have no apparent connection with its cause. We see how a relatively severe neurotic manifestation can appear out of the blue, so to speak, how it can dominate the family's life for a time, only to subside almost spontaneously; and we are reminded of the importance of looking at the whole problem – the child's problem and the family's emotional difficulties – and of attempting to relieve those parental anxieties which are at the root of the pressure which they exert upon the child.

Steven had had hiccough for months, described as being continuous, day and night. His mother said he had cried about it and was ashamed of it, but it had improved with treatment and had been infrequent during the last two months before we saw him. The pediatrician, who suggested his referral to the child guidance clinic, had prescribed amitriptyline and largactil, the latter to be used in the event of a bad attack. How far the credit for the improvement can be attributed to these remedies is a matter of conjecture, but where there is likelihood that a chemical therapy will alleviate a distressing symptom this ought to be used even when psychological measures also are contemplated. In his referral letter the family doctor said that he considered the hiccough was usually due to family crisis and that when he had last seen Steven he was 'hiccuping like mad' and had been brought by his grandmother, who said that the boy's mother was having an attack of nerves and was thrashing him to make him stop the hiccup. Steven was slightly over twelve when he came to see us, his I.Q. was 101 and his school reports were satisfactory. He had been on school trips to the Continent and was full of information about these, but said that he had had to miss this summer's trip because 'my nerves were too bad'. He was a good mixer and had many friends, with whom he tended to be overpossessive.

Steven's mother had divorced his father for desertion and indeed he had not seen his father since before he was two years old. His mother subsequently remarried and this stepfather was kind to the children, although his paternal instincts were poorly developed.

TREATMENT FOR CHILDREN

Steven had largely been brought up by his grandparents, to whom he still had a strong attachment. His mother, attractive, friendly, and fond of her children, was nevertheless sensitive, basically anxious and without insight. Steven had been bottle fed from birth, as there was a suspicion of his mother's having tuberculosis, although this cleared up satisfactorily and soon. Toilet training was begun at six months and was effected without difficulty and seemingly without much stress. The circumstances of father's desertion must have been traumatic to his mother and, indirectly at least, to the children, but Steven was described as being a happy, contented baby. At the age of five he had bronchitis and at seven measles encephalitis, being unconscious for three days. The pediatrician expressed himself as confident that this was not the cause of the hiccough. Returning to school after this illness, he found himself unequal to its educational demands and he had then been sent to a residential school for delicate children, at which he remained for two years until the age of nine. Thereafter he had been able satisfactorily to cope with the requirements of ordinary schooling. His hobbies were said to be cooking, science and sports. Steven's mother had to have a major surgical operation when he was eight, and was in hospital for six weeks, and from this she made a good recovery.

The family's management of the hiccough seemed to have been an odd process of reasoning and experiment. At first they ignored it; they were generous with their presents and the pediatrician mentioned an expensive transistor radio and a bicycle, although these would probably have been given anyway, and then they put him off television, they stopped his sweets, they took his teddy bear away and they smacked him.

It has to be remembered that by the time Steven came to our clinic the severity of the hiccup had greatly diminished and our handling of his case could therefore be regarded as a mopping-up operation. In his session with the doctor he appeared as an inhibited, insecure child, although he warmed up a little during the interview. We wondered if his mother's description of him as a contented baby might conceal the acceptance of a child who was able to absorb the stresses of a broken home, but whose unconscious anxiety reached high pressure in response. Why the outbreak of hiccough took place when it did never became clear to us. In terms of physiology hiccough seems to be an outmoded form of rejection by the stomach of some noxious substance and we saw it in the present instance as a psychological rejection of unimaginative parental attitudes. Steven expressed himself as being reasonably happy at school and contented with his lot at home. His favourite hobby was fishing, which meant sea fishing in the holidays, and he hoped one day to be an air pilot. He gave the impression of being a boy who had not quite come to terms with his difficulties, whether external or unconscious, and the doctor saw his relatively full and active life as being in some part an escape from the contemplation of these problems. Yet it provided a fairly good adjustment to his circumstances despite his recent breakdown into the hiccough.

Steven's mother told the doctor that there had been a recent all-round improvement in Steven's attitude to life and that he was now happier at school than he had been, was getting on well with his sister and did not appear to have any serious problems. She was not without warmth, yet she struck the doctor as having little insight. Every interpretation he made regarding how he saw the family's attitudes and Steven's situation was strongly countered. Yet the relationship the therapist was getting with her was good enough to stand a gentle and meaningful tease, so that when the doctor said kindly to her that he felt she could argue the hind legs off a donkey she smiled and admitted that there was some truth in the statement. In the end he felt that he had been able to get across to this mother, who was anxious to do her level best for her children, something of her son's need to be regarded as a responsible person with his own natural rights and as a developing adult.

Ideally Steven should have had treatment sessions with a view to helping him overcome his inner anxieties and ameliorate the relative insecurity of his social adjustments. Yet where the total of treatment time is limited we have to concentrate largely on those children whose need is imperative. In any case Steven seemed to be already on the way to recovery by his own efforts. It was therefore decided in our case conference afterwards that we could justifiably leave him to progress under his own steam, especially as the therapist felt that his mother's eyes were partly opened to the requirements of the boy's developing personality. Almost five months afterwards our social worker called. The family were all down with 'flu', but apart from this, Steven was well and there had been no recurrence of hiccough. His mother assured her that she would let us know in the event of further difficulty and the social worker felt that the contact between them was sufficiently good to justify reliance on that statement.

CHAPTER XVI

The Later School Years and School Leavers

1. The Later School Years
Children are now in their early teens and are beginning to experience the resurgence of sexual feelings. In some these may already dominate the emotional scene, but there are many whose inhibitions remain strong and whose active heterosexual interest is slow to develop. Even in their case these sensual stirrings are already in existence, at least subconsciously, and these children usually entertain a richer awareness of sexual interest than they are prepared to admit. We may expect emotions to be revealed in therapy a little more readily than in the case of middle school, or latency, children but we still must proceed with caution.

Psychosomatic Illness: A Problem of Growing Up. Violet was fourteen years and four months when she first came to our clinic with the complaint of abdominal pain which she said was frequently severe. She was the elder of two children, her brother being eight years younger than she, and she had an I.Q. of 124. She attended a secondary modern school. The original referral was by the pediatrician to the child guidance clinic of a local authority which shortly afterwards suffered a reduction of its territory, and it was after Violet had attended there for several months that the clinic abruptly ceased to function and she transferred to our clinic. During the early phase of treatment there was great resistance to the acceptance of the symptoms as being of nervous origin, a resistance which Violet's mother reinforced, and had it not been that the symptoms were distinctly painful and that the family doctor and pediatrician both refused to support the desired explanation that there must be an organic cause, she would not have continued to come for treatment.

The mother was an anxious individual who suffered from fits of which we had no diagnosis and for which she took medicine, and was herself currently attending a psychiatric out-patient department. In one of these fits she had dropped Violet at the age of eighteen months.

The child had a skull fracture and was in hospital for ten days, her parents visiting daily. The father expressed much concern regarding his daughter's health, but it was our impression that there was deep-seated stress within the family and that this stemmed to a considerable extent from his resentments and aggressive temperament. Violet was stated to have been a 'normal' child for the first five years of her life and to have been a much-loved baby. She was breast-fed and was weaned at six months, after which it was said that she would eat only chocolate. She walked at ten months, talked at fifteen months and her periods started when she was eleven. She started to have acute attacks of abdominal pain soon after her brother's birth. The pediatrician described these as 'periodic syndrome'. Reports from school had been on the whole good, but with some recent falling off. She wanted success, but applied herself indifferently to the work, while her total achievement was much below her intellectual potential. In her spare time she seemed often to be either entertaining friends or being entertained in their homes, and she would very much have liked to have a regular boy friend, although being afraid of what this might lead to. It was said also that her pain got her out of the need to perform unpleasant duties, a not very surprising attribute of neurotic disability.

When Violet came to us she had already had five treatment interviews at the other clinic and points which came through clearly in the notes were her undue dependence on her parents, her inability to express resentment against her parents and her ambivalent attitude towards boys. In our first session the patient said she was appreciably better than she had been, this bearing out a similar comment in the note of the last interview at the other clinic. How far this was from reality was to be apparent during the months of treatment which were to follow. At this point, however, it was evident that there would be a considerable resistance to further therapy, and after discussing the possibilities with Violet, and then with her and her mother together, the therapist left it to them to decide if they wanted further help and to let him know of their decision.

Three weeks later they returned, without having made an appointment, to say that Violet had been having a lot of pain as well as retching, if not actual vomiting. Her mother added that this was the usual situation before each alternate period. Violet said that there would be no good in coming to the therapist for treatment, that the previous psychiatrist had asked questions, and so forth. She said she had some 'tablets' from the family doctor. The therapist mentioned the possibility, as an alternative to therapy in the clinic, that she might come into hospital for a week when the symptoms were bad or else that we might try to find a place for her in a residential school. This last suggestion the patient turned down flat. Under these circumstances we decided to leave matters in abeyance for a month or two. Almost two months from that day Violet came back with her mother as a matter of urgency because the pains had been severe. The psychiatrist outlined the treatment situation and its possibilities, in great detail, and the patient accepted that something was necessary and she agreed to come.

In her first treatment session she outlined the position and periodicity of this, left-sided, abdominal pain. She spoke of relationships at home which, superficially at least, were good. Her father was out a good deal and she would have liked to have more attention from him, but mother, having had pain herself, was sympathetic. She now had a boy friend and when the pain had recently started when they were at the pictures he had been considerate. She was waking a good deal during the night, she said, but she never had any dreams. Sometimes she had nausea at meals. In the relative silence which followed the doctor suggested that she might paint something, and as she was unwilling to attempt this, he painted a 'butterfly' and Violet accepted that a painting by her might be of assistance to him.

The doctor arranged for Violet to come half an hour early next time in order to paint while he was occupied elsewhere. In actual fact she spent three-quarters of an hour drawing the house on the other side of the street, which was visible through the window, and even then she did not get far with her drawing. The doctor discussed how very shut in her feelings were, as revealed by the poverty of expression in the picture and her slowness in making it. He again asked about dreams, but she said she had none. It was almost impossible to get any verbal expression from Violet and in the next session the therapist spoke about bowel motions, urine, tears and sweat, and thus got to the subject of physiology. From there he talked about menstruation, conception and birth, and finally he said something about the emotional difficulties of boys, who often thought that girls had an easier time socially than did boys. Violet said almost nothing, but seemed to be with the doctor in grasping what he had been saying.

At their next meeting Violet told the therapist that she had been off school for three days because of the pain and that she had gone to the doctor, who gave her medicine. The therapist, reflecting on the drawing of the house over the road, talked of how afraid she was to bring out anything of herself, said he wondered what she was afraid of and went on to explain that she must in some way be afraid of him, seeing that she could say so little to him. She must be afraid, for instance, that he might think badly of her if he knew the thoughts and feelings that were inside her. He spoke of such feelings, sexual ones, aggressive ones, jealousies, and said how these were emotions which could hardly be so bad, as they were natural and as we all shared them. He then happened to ask her how she was sleeping. She told him that she slept with her brother, but that they had been discussing a change round at home whereby she could sleep with her mother and her brother with their father. The therapist discussed this plan with Violet and he led round to such possibilities as that they might alter the arrangements in one of the other rooms so that it could be used as a bedroom for her brother at night. She said that she was bothered about forthcoming exams and she said that her cake had come out well (to her surprise) and that it was to be for her parents' wedding anniversary next month and would be a surprise for them.

In the next session she had to report pains on three evenings. She said that she sometimes went out with her boy friend, that her father was friendly towards her doing so and that he said: 'Don't get into any trouble.' I have often pondered on this working-class propensity to assume that young people will have sexual intercourse unless their parents tell them not to.

The therapist worked round to talk of masturbation. Violet agreed that she understood his meaning and smiled. He discussed her fear of the unknown and of what happened when one was married or in love and had sexual intercourse. He spoke of his belief that she resented not getting enough of her father's interest or of his time. He asked about dreams, but she said she had had none.

In the following session he tried to continue discussing her feelings further, including feelings about himself. Violet said that he, the therapist, had other patients besides herself and she had noticed that he consulted his notes at the beginning of the interview, so that he could not be sufficiently interested in her if he did not remember about her. The therapist had to admit that both these charges were true and that in so far as the second was concerned he did have difficulty in remembering all that he would wish to and that he therefore made a few notes in order to ensure that things were not forgotten. He said how she felt that he did not care sufficiently about her and how, indeed, she had a deep down feeling that neither Dad nor Mum nor anyone really did love her sufficiently. In the next session the talk continued in this vein and the therapist referred to her resentment about the pain – why did *she* have this and not others and boys did not have menstrual difficulties? – but she would not admit to such resentment. As Violet was virtually silent all this time, he had to twist and turn in his suggestions as to how she felt about her various circumstances, and in time he got back to her feeling that he did not really care about her and that she sometimes felt that no one cared. He spoke of her feeling that she was not as good as, or not worth as much as, other girls. In the following week it was of headache that she complained and for most of the time the doctor could get nothing from Violet. As he talked of her feelings she sometimes gave a faint smile and the therapist got a hunch that it was as though her unconscious were saying that the pain was not really just so bad. At the very end of the interview she said that she was totally bored with everything.

During the next session the psychiatrist worked out with Violet how she was hurt by the fact that her father was out too much and did not take sufficient interest in her, although it was difficult to get her to express any feelings whatever. She waited till right at the end of the interview to say that she was having a party on Sunday for her parents' wedding anniversary, for which it will be remembered that she had earlier baked the cake, and she asked him if she should tell her parents beforehand that she was going to do this. Her using the psychiatrist in this way was evidence of a growing, positive relationship with him. At the next session Violet said that the party had gone well and she gave the doctor a piece of the cake which she had brought for him. He spoke of her feeling of not liking herself and Violet said that she thought of herself as being lower than anyone else. The doctor then spoke of resentments, of nasty behaviour, of being ashamed of some parts of our bodies and of feeling guilty about some of the things we did, and he said how all these characteristics of function and episodes of unflattering behaviour were common to all of us. He spoke of some of the qualities of which girls were possibly ashamed, such as body hair, small breasts or a prominent bottom. Violet uttered a very faint 'Yes'. The therapist spoke of how her pains were bound up with bad feelings.

Right at the start of the following session Violet burst into tears, buried her head in her hands and said she was fed up. Then for forty minutes she said not another word, while the therapist talked of her feelings. Eventually she said she was fed up, no one cared about her, she was bored, especially of going to Blackpool for the holidays, but her father would not agree to any change. In the hall, on rejoining her mother at the end of the session, she burst into tears once more, put her head on the therapist's shoulder and her arm round him and remained in this position for several minutes. Her mother tried to say comforting things and Violet replied that she wanted to die and that they could kill her. During this episode she developed an obvious attack of abdominal colic.

Because of what had come to light the therapist was anxious to meet Violet's father and he came in the week following what has just been described. This was a cordial interview in which it was possible to discuss, among other things, what alterations he felt he could make in the holiday plans: he was willing to make changes, although not to go exactly where Violet wanted. Another meaningful thing he said was that right from her brother's birth she had felt she was being pushed out and that nowadays she was very desirous that her little brother should need her to do things for him and that she liked when he asked her to do things and when he ordered her about. About this time mother told our social worker that father was very obsessional in his insistence on certain formalities and that he was thus a difficult man. In the interview which followed Violet talked more freely than usual on various matters and after she had left the therapist at the end she returned to ask if her mother should come to see the social worker the following week. The therapist believed that the real reason for coming back was in order to reassure herself of his interest in her.

In the next interview she said that her father was 'tough'. There had been an opportunity to arrange a holiday in the Channel Islands, but she doubted if he would agree. She went on to say that about the time of her first coming to our clinic there had been a bad row between mother and father, so much so that mother went to see a friend who agreed to take her and the children in to live. Apparently they did not actually go and things had been easier since. Violet also raised a matter which the doctor had discussed much earlier, namely the possibility of her being happier if she could go to a residential school. Now, for the first time, she said she would be agreeable to going, although she still was not keen, and the matter was not further pursued, partly for this reason and partly owing to the great difficulty in getting boarding-school places at her age. The next interview showed father up in a more favourable light, because when Violet had wakened in the night with pain he had gone and got her a hot bottle which cured the pain through a combination perhaps of the heat from the bottle and the warmth of paternal love. Having told of this, Violet said not another word for the rest of the interview, and it was left to the therapist to discuss emotional meanings, such as that of the hot-water bottle incident. He also said something about father's own human limitations and the hardships which he must have suffered and which were at the root of his sometimes difficult attitudes.

When the next session came round Violet said she was much better. She had fallen out, she said, with her boy friend on account of his mother's pressure on him. The therapist might have discussed what had been the unconscious purpose of this relationship, for example in providing her with love, social status among coevals and the fantasy of future security, and whether it was perhaps less necessary to have this boy friendship now that there had been an improvement in her situation at home. When it came to the session after this Violet still said that she was a little better, although she had had some pain in the previous week-end. She mentioned the relaxation treatment that her mother was having for her nervousness. The doctor talked about feelings – love, hatred, aggression, feelings against oneself and suicide. To some of this Violet assented, once she said 'No', but mostly she was silent. When eventually the doctor said it was time to say 'Good-bye' – i.e. the end of the interview – she burst into tears, said no one believed her pains were real, that her mother and father did not believe her, and she said with special feeling that her father had been out on Saturday evening, that when he came in she had had pains and that he only said that it was nonsense and that she must get better herself. She went on to say that Daddy did not love her and did not care and that Mummy did not believe her. The doctor spoke about her interpretation of her father's unfortunate attitudes and of how much of her feeling about his not caring was really not quite true of him, but was her own feeling of herself as not being worth caring for. He discussed her father as not understanding rather than as not caring. Violet made no response to this, but when she did say 'Good-bye' to the doctor she appeared to be reassured and happier. In the session which followed this one she claimed to have maintained her improvement, although she was still not entirely free from the pains.

At the next session Violet said she was much happier and she appeared to be happy. She said a little more about the difficulties which had caused her and her boy friend to separate and she did not appear to be at all upset by the experience. It had also been arranged that she would go on holiday with a girl friend and she was pleased about this. The therapist felt that by this time Violet's condition was a good deal more stable than it had been and that she should now be able to carry on on her own with, perhaps, occasional help from him. He therefore suggested coming once more in three weeks' time and subsequently at her own choice. He promised also to get in touch with the youth employment officer, as questions had arisen as to what Violet would do once she left school. She returned after three weeks wearing a new costume and appearing to be fairly happy, but she still did not have much to say.

Some of the adolescents whom we meet in their middle-school years have problems which largely concern practical issues and the emotional urges to which they give rise, and it may then be our appropriate task to assist in straightening these out, without much reference to the deeper causes of the emotions involved.

Behaviour Disorder Reactive to School Stress. We were asked to see Julian when he was almost fourteen on account of behaviour disorder at school. This involved fighting, threatening people with a knife, shaking his fist at teachers and other children and pulling distorted faces. He felt that he was being treated unjustly and was so constantly on the defensive that he was ready to respond aggressively at the first hint of criticism. Within the stressful relationship which had developed, his teachers appeared to be comparably ready to nip in the bud any false step that he might take. His headmaster actually suspended him from school shortly before we were able to see him and until the clinic should have made as assessment. Julian was the fourth of five children and intelligence testing gave him an I.Q. of 99.

So far as we were aware, the parents' marriage was a happy one, but as we never were able to acquire an intimate understanding of this family's life it may have been less good than was claimed. Father appeared to be something of a nonentity in the society in which he moved and to play a relatively insignificant part even in his own family. Mother always appeared to us as displaying an average amount of concern regarding her son's difficulties and both school and clinic regarded the parents as being co-operative. The therapist's conclusion was, however, that they had failed to give to their children a stable example of good family management and that they were weak and in some degree lacking in responsibility.

Julian was artificially fed from birth – we did not discover the reason for this – and was described as a happy and contented baby. Toilet training was started early, but no outstanding difficulties appeared to have been encountered. Almost three years before Julian first came to see us his mother had been in hospital for three days following a cycle accident and the children were able to go and wave to her through the window. This little story appears to speak for a happy family relationship. Julian had a number of interests. He kept birds and showed them, he was interested in historic buildings which they would visit by car as a family, he collected stamps, had camped, was a member of a youth club and had a number of friends. He had also been in trouble with the police for minor offences and was on probation for a time. His parents were satisfied with his standard of behaviour at home; he wished to get on well with people, but he was a boy who needed to be coaxed into compliance and who found it difficult to conform if he did not get his own way.

Julian, then, came to us under the cloud of having been suspended

TREATMENT FOR CHILDREN

from school, and the most striking thing about him in the first interview was that, under these circumstances, he was ready to be flippant. He said that he was happy and this, in many respects, was true. He claimed a good relationship with his mother, but said that his father was inclined to be critical. He explained the school situation from his own viewpoint, saying that the masters picked on him. Recently in an exam the master had said that a boy should put up his hand if he did not understand the meaning of any of the words used. When Julian put his hand up the master just looked at him facetiously. Julian therefore had to ask one of the other boys and for this he was sent out of the room. He said that he had good friends of both sexes, but it seemed to the doctor that he might be quite difficult to live with. The doctor decided that he must try to get to know Julian better and to help him in that way, but it was touch and go whether he would agree to continue to come. In the event he did.

The doctor phoned the headmaster, who said that Julian became white with rage. He said he would do what he could in the Easter holidays which were close at hand, and would get in touch with the school again at the end of that period. In his next interview with Julian he discussed the boy's need, if insulted, to respond with rage. He asked about life at home, and it appeared that Julian and his older siblings managed to tolerate each other, but with occasional outbursts. Father would let his feelings build up inside himself and would then explode and Julian would run off if he felt the immediate temperature was too hot. Mother would get annoyed if she came to the end of her tether, but he generally got on well with her. Julian brought some of his drawings to this interview – of girls, except for one which was of a boy with a koala bear – and these depicted the very important, loving side of his nature. In the next interview he told of being beaten up some time back at the club and of a row at home with his brother, but they were also fond of each other and his brother would help him to punish the boy who had hurt his nose. This was apparently the pattern of a fairly stable family life, and again we may stress the importance in therapy of attempting to grasp what are the dynamics of the family's emotional life and of doing what is possible to facilitate the cohesion of its members. Julian agreed to come next week, for the therapist's sake, although it would be in the school holiday. Subsequent interviews followed a similar pattern and at one point Julian spoke of his fondness for walking with a pack on his back and of the chances of the army as a career. At the end of the holidays he returned to school.

Not long after this Julian's form-master came to see the therapist and in a cordial conversation he provided further evidence of how impossibly aggravating Julian was. It was decided to allow him to be largely free of the classroom and to act as messenger to the school secretary, a lady with whom he got on well. He continued to attend the clinic regularly and on one occasion he paid the therapist the compliment of drawing his portrait on the blackboard in colour. We had an enquiry from his former probation officer, who had heard of the present difficulties and who retained an affectionate interest in Julian. Then, one morning Julian came into the clinic and said that the form-master had said to him: 'If you leave me alone, I shall leave you alone.' Julian said he had therefore flatly ignored the form-master – he had taken what he had said quite literally! The form-master had responded, Julian said, by taking him by the lapels and shaking his fist at him. The therapist tried to get Julian to see that he had been unfair in taking his form-master's words in this manner, but after the matter had been discussed at some length he realized that Julian was by now so much out for the form-master's blood that it would be unsafe to let him return to school in the meantime. He therefore gave a certificate to excuse him for several weeks on medical grounds.

The therapist considered that a conference between Julian, the form-master and himself would hold some hope of reconciliation and he was able to arrange this. The master was extraordinarily generous in the length to which he was willing to go towards an apology and the details of what had been done and said were not argued, it being just accepted that there had been this severe clash of feeling. It was far more difficult to get Julian to yield anything of his resentment and he accepted the reconciliation with reluctance. The therapist was still afraid to let him return to school and he bent his efforts towards arranging a residential school place for him. Julian's co-operation in this was uncertain, that of the school health service was indifferent and we were never able to find a suitable residential place.

We invited Julian to come to camp for nine days in the summer holidays, at his parents' expense subsidized by the social worker's clinic fund, and he accepted. This passed off successfully, but one incident may deserve mention. On the Sunday we expected the boys to attend church and three boys, all from the clinic, said they did not want to go or would not go. One of these, of course, was Julian. In the case of the other two the officer commanding simply said that he felt they had better parade to church with the others and this they did. Knowing of Julian's circumstances and Julian being a little older, he took a different line, explaining that there was need for help with the digging of a latrine pit (which was, in fact, the case) and that he would like Julian to help with this. Julian willingly put in an hour or more at strenuous digging.

During several interviews in the autumn Julian behaved like a child of six years old, playing with toys, running around the room, trying to speak into the telephone and talking to the therapist in the patronizing manner which young children occasionally adopt. This was clearly a regression to an earlier phase of development and showed his need to be allowed to be a child and to be accepted and loved for what he was. On another occasion he said to the doctor, spontaneously and with nothing leading up to the remark: 'I'm not a bad boy. I don't go about hitting teachers.' In the late autumn and early winter there was a change of psychiatrist in the clinic, and although Julian had been prepared for this he arrived one day, early in this period, to complain bitterly of two school prefects who had set upon him. He was resentful about the change of therapist, but after half an hour of violent and angry talk he calmed down and consented to come to see the new psychiatrist if he wanted help.

The usual clinic psychiatrist returned to find a situation whereby Julian was excluded from school by official edict, he still had six months to run of compulsory schooling according to law and as the law precluded his taking a job because he was of school age there was little for him to do day after day. Here was a situation calculated to invite delinquency, but appeals from the clinic to the authorities to make an exception to the rule against employment were met by the ineffectual response that they were not legally permitted to do so. These months were from the therapist's point of view the most difficult, and weekly visits to the clinic were a doubtful bastion against the risks of the remaining hours of idleness to a boy of Julian's temperament. During this time Julian's elder brother was sent by the magistrates to an approved school, but Julian lasted out this difficult time without getting on the wrong side of the police. There was one incident of drunkenness, but this was a Christmastime affair and took place while the usual therapist was still away from the clinic. The Court appearance took place after his return and its imminence was mentioned only at the very end of the interview, the therapist having been told nothing about the event. The therapist took the matter seriously because of Julian's precarious hold on respectability, arranged for his representation by a solicitor and attended the Court himself. In the event a small fine satisfied society's outraged conscience.

This longish period – sixteen months – of therapy ended abruptly with the termination of the school year, because Julian made no further approach to the clinic. At our written request, however, he paid us a visit a short time ago. He was working, he had much pleasure in his new motor cycle which he showed to us and he appeared to be happy and to be satisfactorily adjusted in his everyday affairs. His adolescent urge to be independent and his need to break away from the trammels of authority, which had at times encompassed him so uncomprehendingly, appear to me as sufficient explanation for the cleanness of the break he made with us.

What kind of therapy was this? At only one point did it seem to probe any depth, namely the short period during which Julian's behaviour in the clinic regressed to a childhood level. The remainder might seem to have been superficial and, however necessary, little more than an *ad hoc* manipulation of whatever happened to be the immediate stress. Yet in the writer's view this is correctly to be regarded as a course of analytically orientated treatment. At every turn judgments had to be made, whether in the clinic, at camp or in regard to relationships with adult authority figures, based on a grasp of the boy's feelings and his likely, unconsciously motivated responses. Even more subtly, his awareness that the therapist valued him as a person provided a necessary emotional support during this period of psychological instability, and of bewilderment at the force of relationship difficulties into which he was running, but which he could not understand. The strength of this relationship was nowhere more evident than in the resentment he displayed at the therapist's desertion of him when he visited the clinic during the therapist's absence.

II. *The School Leavers*

Piaget says somewhere that adolescence is characterized by the onset of reflective thought. It is a time of conflicting needs at the emotional level and in the area of social relationships many adolescents are so estranged from their parents that life at home has become almost untenable and a number have been forced out of their homes and have virtually nowhere to go. Those who go to work are aware of the new-found power which the possession of money affords. Some are attracted by the excitement of gang loyalties and inter-gang warfare in our big towns – as one teenager said to the writer, this is more fun than football or snooker. Others again, those who are introverted or neurotic, are torn by uncertainties or by a sense of failure and feel shut off from the community. Their requirements from us are different from those of children and it has even been claimed that child psychiatrists do not understand adolescents and that the 'adolescent' psychiatrist is an animal *sui generis*. Yet until adequate provision is made in special clinics or competent counselling services it will be most regrettable if – as indeed often happens now – the staffs of child guidance clinics desert school leavers just because they have left school. Someone with the requisite understanding is needed who will make a commitment to the adolescent and will stand by him, if need be for several years, even if interviews are infrequent and need not always be lengthy.

Problems of an Established Neurosis in Later Teen Years. Justin first came to see us six weeks before his birthday when he would be seventeen, having been referred by his doctor to the adult psychiatric clinic, where the psychiatrist considerately passed him over to us. His symptoms were that, beginning five years before he came to us and just before the age of twelve, he had attacks of hearing voices and hallucinations of nightmarish type followed by depression and despondency. There was also some temporary disorder of body image. He was the eldest of three children. His I.Q. was 111 and he got a place in a grammar school, but as this proved rather much for him he was sent to a secondary modern school when the family moved home. He was then aged twelve years four months, but the family moved twice more while he was still at school. He was therefore at three secondary modern schools in each of which he was happy. We assessed his personality as being introverted and introspective, he lacked self-confidence, he suffered considerably from ideas of reference and hypochondriacal anxieties were prominent. He was also prone to phases of depression and to migrainous attacks. He told us that some of these symptoms had been present long before the age of twelve.

Justin had been taken to another child guidance clinic round about his twelfth birthday; he saw the psychologist and two psychiatrists and prognoses of varying degrees of severity were made. An E.E.G. at that time was suggestive of 'a liability to disorders having an epileptic element' and another done two months later showed 'some improvement'. Two Rorschach tests were inconclusive and showed 'suspicion of bizarreness and emotional disturbance but insufficient bizarreness (contamination) to indicate schizophrenia', which diagnosis had been made by one of the psychiatrists. That clinic was short of psychiatric time and Justin did not have any treatment there. At the age of fifteen he passed the examination for the Army Apprentice School, to which he went for ten months, but as he was very unhappy there, he was discharged. He then got a job as projectionist in a local cinema and he was doing this work satisfactorily when he came to see us.

Justin's mother said that he got attacks of shivering after going to bed and became very scared before falling asleep. He was easily hurt and she found him a difficult boy to live with. Because she noticed that he had frequent erections she suspected a sexual problem and he was very jealous of the sister next younger than he.

Justin's father was on war service during his early childhood, so that he saw little of him. He was described as irresponsible, the marriage was not a happy one and Justin afterwards complained of his drunkenness and waste of money. There had been a number of instances of unhappy marriages among older relatives and the sex life of the present marriage had been disappointing. Father had finally left two years before Justin came to us, but he continued to send a small weekly income for the children.

As regards etiology we assessed the home circumstances as having played an appreciable part, but we considered that there was also some constitutional loading as seen, for example, in the E.E.G. It was considered that some of the attacks were probably migrainous and that an epileptic element was a possibility. While, however, some of the symptoms were suggestive of other than a purely emotional cause, this was inconclusive.

At the initial interview Justin said that he did not feel well. The attacks, as have been described, came on mostly at night and he felt very nervous, but once he got to sleep he slept well and he felt well afterwards. He said he was very shy and had neither hobbies nor friends, except for one girl whom he thought he had last seen about a week ago, but he liked his work as projectionist. He thought that an accident at the age of eleven had been the cause of the trouble. The doctor asked him what he would like to do in life and Justin said he hoped to work his way up in his present industry, but as nothing was said about making a home of his own the doctor said: 'You're not going to get married?' He replied: 'If I can.' The doctor outlined how the symptoms were not due to the accident which he had mentioned, but arose from his inability to face up to the stresses of living. Justin partially accepted this.

The first treatment interview was two months later and on this occasion the patient said his symptoms had improved, but that he was still moderately depressed. It came out that he was suspicious of people's intentions and found it difficult to trust anyone. With his girl friend he had difficulty in being spontaneous in expression or naturally free in behaviour and the therapist discussed the origins of these problems from the difficulties he had experienced as a child. In the second treatment interview he outlined his symptoms similarly, expressed his fears of another breakdown and when asked about his feelings towards other people he said that he thought that people did not have the intelligence that he had and that he treated them accordingly. The therapist explained how he was, in fact, feeling towards other people both that he was very inferior and that he was very superior. He said how difficult we found it to become the same as others – neither much better nor much worse – and how Justin had either to be unworthy and unequal to others or else he must be supreme and contemptuous of them. Justin told the doctor how readily jealous he was of any potential rival in his own territory and how ambitious he was for his own success.

The next two or three interviews were similarly devoted to his personality attitudes and in speaking of these he displayed a fair measure of insight. He told that he was having an interview for work in one of the large retail stores and he then went on to say that he was doing a good deal of reading about the Second World War and that he had a special interest in this from the German point of view. He said that he was expressing his own hostility in his thoughts about war and that he imagined himself as the general conquering country after country. He felt that anyone who was not with him was against him. The therapist put in the remark that these sorts of ambitious feelings were common to a great many of us and how, if we were honest with ourselves, we hated and even wanted to destroy others who were rivals. He went on to speak of Justin's father and his aggressiveness and of how the assertive drives of Justin's childhood had clashed with his father's personality. A stressful rivalry situation must have arisen when his father returned from military service. Haffner has recently pointed out that adolescents in treatment need to be put in touch with their infancy, of the experiences of which there is a good deal of unconscious acting out in adolescence.[106] Justin said that football provided him with an outlet, that he was anxious to win fame and that prowess in sport sometimes afforded the opportunity he needed to excel over others.

Justin at this time spoke also of the reverse side of the coin. He was upset by what people said about him, if he were teased or if anyone were sarcastic. He thought that his hostile attitudes ought to be altered and he was worried because, as he believed, his co-ordination in athletics was impaired whereas in his school days he had excelled in sporting events; and he was afraid that the knock he had had on the forehead long ago might have made him defective in some way. He said he could not trust himself. He remembered that, when he was nine or ten, his mother made him go to bed earlier than the other children of the neighbourhood, that this made him feel inferior, and that once when he did not come in she gave him a bad thrashing with a stick. In one of the interviews he said he had been to a dance, had almost enjoyed it, though he did not dance himself, and that he felt a little more confident. A week later he described an attack of severe frontal headache which, apart from its being bilateral, had several features of migraine. He said that he was having these attacks about every six months. Although the therapist did not mention epilepsy, it came out that Justin was afraid of this and that he had a widespread fear of mental illness.

Later on he began to talk about his earlier life at home and he said that he thought that this background must have been an important cause of his present attacks of anxiety and depression. He spoke of his father's drinking, of his failure to help his mother and of his eventual desertion. His father's feckless spending had resulted in his mother having to go out to work, as a result of which Justin had felt neglected. On one occasion he had called his father 'a silly old clown' and had been rebuked by his mother for this measure of defiant contempt. He recollected how anxious he used to be at school and how he had pled with his mother not to make him go. He remembered that he had used to produce a pain by contracting some part of his body as an excuse for being allowed to stay at home. By the time he told of these events he had been coming regularly for three and a half months to the clinic; he had recently obtained a new job in which he was happy, and although he continued to feel dependent on coming to see the therapist, he was considerably better adjusted to his environment all round.

In the following few weeks he had one mild relapse with headache, arising in part out of association of ideas in a film, as a result of which he wondered if he could have a cerebral tumour. He had an interesting dream about snakes, the sexual symbolism of which gave the therapist an opening to talk of Justin's anxieties in this area, but the details were, unfortunately, not committed to paper at the time and cannot be recalled now. Sexual matters had not figured prominently in discussions up to this time, largely on account of the immaturity of Justin's emotional responses and his narcissistic anxieties, which had dominated the field of therapeutic enquiry. It was agreed that interviews should be less frequent and by the end of the ninth month of treatment Justin was so well that the decision was taken to stop treatment, with, of course, the proviso that the therapist would like to see him again if need arose. He had at this time three months to go until his birthday when he would be eighteen. He came in just before his birthday and once more six weeks afterwards. He continued to feel well.

It was twenty months later than Justin came to say that he had not been so well of late. He had had an attack of headache accompanied by tingling, disturbance of ocular accommodation which could have been at a mental rather than organic level, and various paraesthesiae, followed by depression. The paraesthetic symptoms had recurred on one or two occasions and the therapist considered that it would be sound policy to ask the neurologist to have a look at him. This was arranged and an E.E.G. also was done, but the findings gave him an entirely clean bill of health. Certain emotional difficulties also were distressing him. Not only did he feel lacking in confidence but he was concerned because he was occasionally picking violent quarrels. He was by this time going with a girl friend and he was finding that when the pleasure of being with her was becoming intense something from inside him came up to stop it. During this and the next session these issues were so far as possible explored, but two months later there was evidence of so much anxiety, along with bizarre symptoms, that the therapist prescribed chlorpromazine. Analytically oriented therapy was not resumed, but the drug appeared to be effective in that there was an appreciable abatement in the severity of the symptoms.

A family circumstance obtruded itself during this period in that Justin's mother got in touch with the social worker because of her distress at finding that the sister next to Justin was pregnant at the age of fifteen. Our social worker dealt adequately with this matter. It is unlikely that the affair could have played other than a minor part in originating the recrudescence of his neurosis from which Justin suffered at this time.

From then onwards Justin continued to come in occasionally to see the therapist for a further three years and during all that time he seemed gradually to gain self-confidence and to grow in psychological strength. At the time of his twenty-first birthday he wrote a chatty and interesting letter and at the time of his last visit he appeared very well and was able to inform us that he was branch manager of a firm in the south-east of England and many miles from his home. His continuing relationship with the clinic had now lasted for five and a half years and it is a contribution of this size that we must sometimes be prepared to make if we are to give to young people in their immediate post-school years the help that some of them need.

Conclusion

Scant attention has been paid in these pages to what we may call the non-analytical forms of approach to child guidance. We have alluded to the absolute importance, for some cases, of an environment away from home in the residential school for maladjusted children or the hospital unit, but in these therapy is founded largely on relationship formation and this must, in its turn, rest upon an understanding of children and their needs. Neither religious indoctrination nor any form of training, unless the adults concerned can love children and can put the children's emotional requirements above considerations of traditional behaviour or even of ethics, are likely to be of much value in solving the problems of childhood nervousness or adolescent maladjustment. To offer the love of God, which is intangible, to children from whom the milk of human kindness has been withheld may come dangerously near to cynicism.

Hypnosis, behaviour therapy and drugs are scientific forms of treatment to which we have alluded only briefly. This is so because of the conviction that in childhood at least recovery from neurosis of any kind will depend upon improved relationship formation and upon an enhanced ability on the child's part to understand himself and to see the meaning of his existence in association with the environment. It is necessary that the therapist should give to the child his time and a part of himself, and that he should have a genuine sympathy and a caring attitude towards him. We may usefully learn to be content to follow our child patient in the latter's use of the therapeutic time available to him, and only sometimes to employ a steering hand towards this or that activity or subject of conversation. We do need to learn to see meanings beneath the surface of what the child says or does, or does not do, and the value of interpretive comment is irreplaceable. Our object is to learn about our children from themselves and to pass back to them, in forms that they can assimilate, what we have learned.

FOR FURTHER READING

Aichorn, A., *Wayward Youth*, 1935, Viking Press, N.Y.
Allen, F. H., *Psychotherapy with Children*, 1947, Kegan Paul, London.
Bowlby, J., *Child Care and the Growth of Love*, 1953, Penguin, Harmondsworth.
Cary, J., *A House of Children*, 1941, Michael Joseph, London.
Foulkes, S. H., and Anthony, E. J., *Group Psychotherapy*, 2nd edn. 1965, Pelican, Harmondsworth.
Hartley, L. P., *The Shrimp and the Anemone*, 1963, Faber, London.
Haworth, M. R. (ed.), *Child Psychotherapy*, 1964, Basic Books Inc., N.Y. and London.
Howells, J. G. (ed.), *Modern Perspectives in Child Psychiatry*, 1965, Oliver and Boyd, Edinburgh.
Isaacs, S., *Social Development in Young Children*, 1933, Routledge and Kegan Paul, London.
Jackson, L., and Todd, K., *Child Treatment and the Therapy of Play*, 1946, Methuen, London.
Kahn, J. H., and Nursten, J. P., *Unwillingly to School*, 1964, Pergamon Press, Oxford.
Kanner, L., *Child Psychiatry*, 2nd edn. 1948, Blackwell, Oxford.
Lewis, E., *Children and their Religion*, 1962, Stag Books, Sheed and Ward, N.Y.
Rogerson, C. H., *Play Therapy in Childhood*, 1939, Oxford University Press.
Slavson, S. R., *Group Therapy in Children*, 1943, The Commonwealth Fund, N.Y.
Soddy, K., *Clinical Child Psychiatry*, 1960, Baillière, Tindall & Cox, London.
Winnicott, D. W., *The Family and Individual Development*, 1965, Tavistock Publications, London.

NOTES

[1] Cf. p. 34.
[2] Pasamanick, B., Rogers, M. E., and Lilienfeld, A. M., *Amer. J. Psychiat.*, 1956, *112*, 613.
[3] Drillen, C. M., *Develop. Med. Child Neurol.*, 1963, *5*, 3.
[4] Caplan, G., and Bowlby, J., *Health Ed. J.*, Apr. 1948, 5.
[5] Freud, S., *Collected Papers*, Vol. II.
[6] Soddy, K., *Clinical Child Psychiatry*, 1960, London, Baillière, Tindall, & Cox.
[7] The names of 'Charles' and 'Brackenhurst' which we have used to describe this boy and his family are, of course, fictitious ones, as indeed are all the names attributed to patients whose cases are referred to in the text.
[8] Isaacs, S., *Social Development in Young Children*, 1933, London, Routledge & Kegan Paul.
[9] Tavistock Clinic, London, N.W.3.
[10] Perhaps the best account of emotional and intellectual development is that given by Susan Isaacs, *Social Development in Young Children*.
[11] D=doctor.   P=Patient.
[12] This sort of activity is so common in little children as to be a normal concomitant of this stage of development, and if one is to call it 'masturbation' it is tantamount to saying that virtually all little children masturbate. I wished to avoid this, as the term is associated in the minds of most people with genital stimulation to produce orgasm, and in the male emission, as a substitute for sexual intercourse. Nevertheless it is the case that little children derive pleasurable sensations from these activities.
[13] libido: the term coined by Freud to indicate sensual gratification, sensual pleasure or the energy of the sex instinct or pleasure-seeking instinct. It is the crude, sensual desire in which love and sexual feeling have their common origin.
[14] Charles Berg produces a good deal of the evidence in *Deep Analysis*, 1947, London, Allen & Unwin.
[15] Hollingworth, Leta S., *The Psychology of the Adolescent*, New York, Staples Press Ltd., 1937.
[16] pp. 13 et ff.
[17] Cephalhaematoma is a swelling under the scalp caused by extravasated blood.
[18] Bassa, D. M., *Brit. Med. J.*, Sept. 15, 1962.
[19] Kinesthetic and proprioceptive sensations are those of movement and position.
[20] Allen, F. H., and Pearson, G. H. J., *Brit. J. Med. Psychol.*, *8*, 212.
[21] Strabismus is a squint. Pneumoencephalogram is a brain test.
[22] *Lancet*, Oct. 7, 1961, p. 818.
[23] Cf. p. 61.
[24] Creak, E. M., 1963, *Brit. J. Psychiat.*, *109*, 84-9.
[25] Cf. Rimland, B., *Infantile Autism*, 1964, New York, Appleton-Century-Crofts.
[26] This term is used for want of a better one. Cf. p. 56.
[27] Leading article, *Brit. Med. J.*, Oct. 22, 1966, p. 962.

TREATMENT FOR CHILDREN

[28] Kanner, L., *Child Psychiatry*, Blackwell Scientifice Publications, Oxford.
[29] *Lancet*, 1956, June 23, 1005.
[30] Catzel, P., *Brit. Med. J.*, 1965, June 26, 1673.
[31] Soddy, K., *op. cit.*
[32] Cf. p. 45.
[33] Cf. p. 38.
[34] Cf. Rose, p. 214.
[35] Soma is 'body' as distinct from 'mind.'
[36] Atlee, J., *Abdominal Pain in Children*, London, Butterworth.
[37] *Lancet*, 1955, Nov. 26, 1115.
[38] *Lancet*, 1954, Nov. 20, 1063.
[39] Dally, P. J., 1969, *Anorexia Nervosa*, Heinemann.
[40] Balint, M., 1957, *The Doctor, his Patient, and the Illness*, London, Pitman Medical Publishing Company.
[41] Kanner, L., 1948, *op. cit.*
[42] Stalker, H., and Band, D., 1946, *J. Ment. Sci.*, 92, 324.
[43] Jones, R. W., and Tibbetts, R. W., 1959, *J. Ment. Sci.*, 105, 371.
[44] Soddy, K., 1960, *op. cit.*
[45] Barbour, R. F., *et. al.*, 1963, *Brit. Med. J.*, Sept. 28, 787.
[46] Pyloric stenosis is blockage of outlet from the stomach.
[47] Burnett, N. T., 1957, *Brit. Med. J.*, Aug. 3, 301.
[48] Rogers, C. R., 1939, *The Clinical Treatment of the Problem Child*, London, George Allen & Unwin.
[49] Paulett, J. D., and Tuckman, E., 1958, *Brit. Med. J.*, Nov. 22, 1, 267.
[50] Shaffer, D., Costello, A. J., and Hill, I. D., *Arch. Dis. Childh.*, 1968, 43, 665.
[51] Reid, R. S., 1959, paper read before Midland Child Guidance Group.
[52] p. 38.
[53] Anthony, E. J., 1957, *Brit. J. Med. Psychol.*, 30, 146.
[54] Woodmansey, A. C., *op cit., infra*.
[55] Leading article, *Brit. Med. J.*, Oct. 6, 1962.
[56] Bockner, S., *J. Ment. Sci.*, 1959, 1078.
[57] Cf. p. 113.
[58] Corbett, J. A., *et al.*, 1969, *Brit. J. Psychiat.*, 528, 1229.
[59] Soddy, K., *op. cit.*, 214.
[60] Woodmansey, A. C., 1967, Emotion and the Motions, *Brit. J. Med. Psychol.*, 40, 207–23.
[61] Soddy, *op. cit.*, p. 200.
[62] Warin, R. P. *Brit. Med., J.*, 1 Oct., 1960, 1014.
[63] Kahn, J. H., and Nursten, J. P., *Unwillingly to School*, Oxford, Pergamon Press Ltd.
[64] Jung, C. G., *Psychology of the Unconscious*, translated by Beatrice M. Hinkle, M.D., 1915, London, Kegan Paul, Trench, Trubner & Co.
[65] Maclay, D. T., 1962, *The Medical Officer*, 2829, Vol. CVIII, 15, 229.
[66] Hood, J., 1964, *J. Ch. Psychother.*, 1, 2, 7.
[67] *Brit. Med. J.*, Apr. 2, 1960, 1054, *et. seq.*
[68] Bonnard, A., 1960, *Brit. Med. J.*, May 14, p. 1508.
[69] Barbara, D. A. ,1958, *Stammering*, London, Hutchison Med. Pub. *Idem. The Psychotherapy of Stuttering*, 1962, Oxford, Blackwell Sci. Pub.
[70] Hallgren, B., 1950, 'Specific Dyslexia', *Acta Psych. et Neurol.*, supp., 65.
[71] Herman, K., 1959, *Reading Disability*, Copenhagen, Munksgaard.
[72] Davidson, Susannah, H. M., *Personal Communication*.
[73] *Brit. Med. J.*, 1962, Dec. 22, 1665.
[74] Burns, C. L., 1963, *Brit. Med. J.*, Jan. 26, 260.

NOTES

[75] Branch, M., and Cash, A., *Gifted Children*, 1966, London, Souvenir Press.
[76] Cunningham, M. A., *et al.*, 1968, *Brit. J. Psychiat.*, *114*, Barker, P., and Fraser, I. A., *idem.*, 855.
[77] Pearce, J. D. W., 1952, *Juvenile Delinquency*, London, Cassell.
[78] *Brit. Med. J.*, 14 Jan. 1967, Leading Article. *World Medicine*, 7 Mar. 1967.
[79] Maclay, D. T., 1965, *Brit. J. Criminol.*, Jan, 63–76.
[80] Knox, J. S., 1960, *J. Ment. Sci.*, *106*, 1472.
[81] Maclay, D. T., 1960, *Brit. Med. J.*, Vol. I, pp. 186–90.
[82] Doshay, L. J., 1943, *The Boy Sex Offender and his Later Career*, New York, Grune and Stratton.
[83] The term 'approved school' will disappear under the Children and Young Persons Act, 1969.
[84] Cf. Turtle, G., *Over the Sex Border*, 1963, London, Gollancz.
[85] Lewis, E., 1962, *Children and their Religion*, London, Sheed and Ward.
[86] Catterall, R. D., 1965, *The Practitioner*, *195*, 620–7.
[87] The various aspects of the subject are competently handled in *The Successful Stepparent*, by Helen Thomson, 1967, London, W. H. Allen.
[88] p. 177.
[89] Cf. Winnicott, D. W., *The Family and Individual Development*, 1965, p. 135, London, Tavistock Publications.
[90] Cf. Maclay, D. T., 'The Children's Psychiatrist in Court Cases Concerning Adoption', *Child Adoption*, 1969, *57*, 35–8.
[91] Miller, D. K., 1967, *Communication to Second Conference on the Psychiatric Care of the Adolescent Patient*, Southampton University.
[92] Scott, P. D., and Willcox, D. R. C., 1965, *Brit. J. Psychiat.*, III, 865.
[93] Connell, P. H., 1965, *Proceedings of the Leeds Symposium on Behaviour Disorders*, pp. 10–17, Dagenham, May and Baker Ltd.
[94] Solomon, J. C., and Hambridge, G., 'Therapeutic Play Techniques', *Amer. J. Orthopsychiat.*, 1955, XXV, 3, 591.
[95] Bryan, H. S., *Athene*, 1959, IX, 2, 5. Published by S.E.A., 37 Denison House, 296 Vauxhall Bridge Road, S.W.1.
[96] This is the boy mentioned on page 103, whose stammer improved.
[97] Cf. Woodmansey, A. C., 'The Internalization of External Conflict', *Internat. J. Psycho-anal.*, 1966, Vol. 47, Parts 2–3, 349–55.
[98] Foulkes, S. H., and Anthony, E. J., *Group Psychotherapy*, 1957, Penguin Books.
[99] Slavson, S. R., 1943, *An Introduction to Group Therapy*, The Commonwealth Fund and Harvard University Press, New York.
[100] Ginot, H. G., 1961, *Group Psychotherapy with Children*, McGraw-Hill Book. Co. Inc., New York.
[101] Young R. A., *Mental Hygiene*, 1939, XXIII, 241–56.
[102] p. 157.
[103] p. 53.
[104] David Bilbey, Headmaster Shenstone Lodge Residential School, West Bromwich Education Authority, and formerly Headmaster of Bodenham Manor Residential School, Herefordshire.
[105] Cf. pp. 44, 133.
[106] Haffner, C.: Address given to the 1967 Southampton Conference on Treatment of Adolescents.

INDEX

INDEX

Abortion, 125
Access by separated parent, 130
Administration, 26, 206
Adolescence, 46, 138, 172
Adoption, 129
Affectionless children, 121
Agarophobia, 181
Age of children, 30, 134
Aggression, 37, 77, 114
Alopecia, 99, 207
Anal phase, 37
Analysis, 35, 44
Anorexia nervosa, 79
Anoxia, 14
Anxiety, 64, 196
Arithmetic, 105
Arson, 115
Asthma, 80
Attitudes, of parents, 39
   of therapist, 44
   to therapist, 134, 166
Autism, 56

Backwardness, 106, 142
Balloon bursting, 151
Bed-wetting, 83
Behaviour, conforming, 35, 44, 50
   disorder, 112, 225
   therapy, 60, 72, 235
Bell, electric, 85, 88
Bereavement, 50, 76, 127
Birth, 12, 33
Birthday cards, 159
Blackboard, 164
Blood, 156
Brain damage, 14, 51
Breast abscess, 13, 99
   feeding, 34
Breath holding, 71

Bronchitis, 34
Burning accidents, 52

Camp, 173, 227
Case Summary, 18
Castration anxieties, 41
Cerebral palsy, *see* Spastic disorder
Child care officer, 22, 27
Children and Young Persons Act, 239
Clumsy children, 109
Colitis, 93
Communication, 24, 26, 60
Compulsions, 72
Concentration, 46, 51
Conference, 27
Confidence, 19, 234
Congenital abnormalities, 62, 115
Constipation, 38, 89
Co-operation, 206
Coprophagy, 93
Counselling, 60, 63
Courts, 28, 121, 130
Cretinism, 13
Croup, 71
Crushes, 49, 125
Cuddling, 34
Custody, 130

Deafness, 55
Defaecation, 37, 88
Defences, 38, 50
Delinquency, 77, 114, 139
Denial, 38
Depression, 76, 117, 145
Destructiveness, 65, 112
Development, 33
Diagnosis, 11, 13, 17
Diary, 47

243

Disabilities, 52
Discussion, 27, 29
Displacement, 38, 193
Divorce, 127
Doctor, family, 1, 13
Doll, 148, 149
Drama, 151
Drawing, 153, 164
Dreams, 98, 133
  daydreams, 47
Drugs, 16, 52, 55, 69, 75, 77, 85, 93, 95, 109, 113, 215, 235
Drug taking, 130
Dyslexia, 104

Early school years, 187
Eating, 47, 69
Electric convulsion therapy (E.C.T.), 77
Eczema, 14, 16, 94
Education authority, 29, 107
Educational subnormality, 107
Ego, 166
Electro-encephalogram (E.E.G.), 55, 62
Electra complex, 41
Emissions, seminal, 47
Encephalitis, 53
Encopresis, 38, 88, 113
Enuresis, 83
Environment, 11, 17
Epilepsy, 7, 54
Escape, 138, 141, 144
Excretory functions, 37, 211
Exposure, indecent, 118, 162
Extroversion, 142, 166

Fainting, 71
Fairy tales, 45
Family, 8, 20, 204
Fantasy, 38, 46
Father, 22, 50, 93
  avenging, 41, 178
Fears, 41, 72, 205
  of separation, 65
Feeding, 12, 34
  bottle, 34, 151, 191

  breast, 34
Feelings, 156, 186, 191
Fire, 149
Food, 35
Free association, 133
Friends of child guidance clinic, 179
Frustration, 14, 34, 135

Games, 148
Gangs, 50
Gastro-enteritis, 34
Genital phase, 38, 134
Gifted children, 110
Gilles de la Tourette syndrome, 93
Group, 50, 170
Growing-up, 47, 71
Guilt, 38, 47, 119

Hair pulling, 70
Hallucinations, 61, 230
Handicapped children, 52
Happy, making child, 132, 136
Hare lip, 52
Headache, 79
Head banging, 16, 70
Herd instinct, 44
Heredity, 14, 115
Hiccough, 215
Home, residential, 129
Homosexual urges, 49, 124
Hospital, 51, 60
Housing, 180
Hunches, 31, 210
Hyperkinesis (hyperactivity), 52, 62
Hypnosis, 82, 85
Hypsarrhythmia, 62
Hysteria, 55, 65

Idealism, 48
Illnesses, 13
Imaginative talking, 179, 200
Immigrant children, 114
Incestuous desires, 38
Industrialization, 19, 39
Infancy, 232
Influences, 102
Inhibition, 136, 178

INDEX

Intellect, 33
Intercourse, 46
Internalized neurosis, 19, 169, 196
Interpretation, 44
Interviews, combined, 170
   frequency of, 59, 134, 139
   missed, 202
Introjection, 41
Introversion, 142, 166

Jealousy, 27, 43
Jerky movements, 70

Kernicterus, 14

Laryngismus stridulus, 71
Latency, 43, 137
Later school years, 218
Later teen years, 229
Learning, 33
Left-handedness, 106
Libido, 39
Local authority, 29
Love, 35, 50, 116
Lying, 115

Maladjustment, 90, 174
Masturbation, 39, 124, 134
Materialism, 19, 50, 116
Meanings, 64, 69, 133
Menstruation, 47, 156
Mental deficiency, 13, 70
   subnormality, 106
Middle school years, 196, 204
Migraine, 95
Milestones of growth, 13, 33
Mirror-writing, 106
Mixing, social, 207
Modelling, 150
Money, 179
Mongolism, 13
Mother, 21, 60
   therapy for, 26, 52, 192
   out at work, 20, 116
Motivation, 117
Motor cars, taking away, 115
Muscular co-ordination, 57, 109

Nail-biting, 70, 211
Narcissism, 49
Nightmares, 68
Night terrors, 69
Note-taking, 221

Obesity, 69
Obsessional illness, 38, 72, 153
Oedema, 204
Oedipus complex, 39, 41, 163
Operant conditioning, 60
Oral phase, 33
Organic states, 13, 51, 62
Overeating, 69

Pain, abdominal, 64, 78, 218
Painting, 32, 153, 220
   bringing to clinic, 163, 208
Parents, 20, 52
   foster, 121, 129
   loss of, 127
   step, 127
Pediatrics, 62, 82
Periodic syndrome, 78
Petit mal, 7, 54
Phallic phase, *see* Genital phase
Phenylketonuria, 13
Phobia, 46, 96, 180
Physical contact, 210
   examination, 13, 62
   factors, *see* Organic
Physiology, 216, 220
Play, 47, 132, 141
   in relation to low intelligence, 106, 142
   situations, 150
   therapy, 106, 132
Polymorph-perverse feelings, 49
Pregnancy, 12, 125
Pre-school years, 134, 178
Probation officer, 27, 117, 227
Problem, nuclear, 11, 133
   working out of, 132
Projection, 38
Prostitution, 115
Psychiatrist, 52, 122, 177
Psychoanalysis, *see* Analysis

245

Psychologist, 12, 17, 121
Psychopath, 34, 121
Psychosis, 55
Psychosomatic illness, 78, 215, 218
Puerperium, 12
Punch-ball, 151
Punishment, 25, 42, 114
   talion, 42
Puppetry, 151
Pyknolepsy, 54

Questions, 144, 179, 208

Rationalization, 213
Reaction formation, 38, 72
Reading disability, 104, 119
Referral, 11
Regression, 38, 43, 228
Rejection, 20, 34, 116
Relationships, 107, 166, 204
Relatives, 12, 60, 181
Religion, 127, 139, 235
Repression, 41, 44, 183
Reserve, see Inhibition
Residential treatment, 92
   home, 129
Resistance, 178
Rocking, rolling, banging, 70
Rubella, 14

Sand tray, 103, 141
Schizoid states, 50, 61
Schizophrenia, 56, 230
School, approved, 122, 177
   change of, 98, 101
   leavers, 229
   medical officer, 11, 97
   phobia, 96, 162
   residential, 98, 174
   special, 58, 107
Self-gratification, 33, 37
Separation, 13
Sex instruction, 45, 199, 209
Sexual offences, 118
Shyness, 136
Sibling jealousy, 43, 186
Silence, 178
Sleep, 15, 75

Sleep walking, 68
Social worker, 12, 22, 177
Soiling, 38, 88
Spastic disorder, 53
Speech difficulty, 100
   therapist, 101
Splitting of personality, 38
Spoilt child, 13, 207
Stammer, 101, 145, 154
Stealing, 115, 116
Step-parents, 127
Subnormality, see Mental subnormality
Sucking, 36, 70, 192
Suckling, 15, 37
Suicide, 77
Summary, 17
Super-ego, 41, 163
Swearing, 93, 115
Symptoms, 12, 64

Taboo, 46, 110
Teacher, 12, 26, 227
Teaching, remedial, 98, 106
Temper tantrums, 114
Test, apperception, 188
Therapist, attitude of, 60, 133, 169
   bad, 45, 163
   faith in, 166
   fear of, 139, 149, 162
   problems of, 133, 213
Thumb sucking, 70
Tics, 92
Toilet training, 38, 89
Tongue sucking, 70
Toxaemia of pregnancy, 14
Toys, 141, 148
Transference, 138, 170
   counter, 133
Trans-sexuality, 125
Transvestism, 120
Treatment, ending of, 213
   in-patient, 60, 92
   of mother, see Mother
Truancy, 114
Trust, 26, 53, 166
Truth, 115

INDEX

Unconscious, 25, 31
Urination, 191
Urticaria, 94, 204

Venereal disease, 126
Vomiting, 79, 95

Wandering, 114

War, 80
Water, 148
Weaning, 12
Word blindness, 104
'Working class', 20, 23, 191

Y chromosome, 115
Young children, 13, 21

247